The Crisis Team

Julian Lieb, M.B., B.Ch.

Instructor in Psychiatry, Yale University
School of Medicine,
Chief Psychiatrist, Depression Research Unit,
Consultant, Medication, Support and
Rehabilitation Unit,
Connecticut Mental Health Center,
New Haven, Connecticut

Ian I. Lipsitch, M.D.

Department of Psychiatry, Yale University
School of Medicine,
New Haven, Connecticut

Andrew Edmund Slaby, M.D.

Department of Psychiatry, Yale University
School of Medicine,
New Haven, Connecticut

The Crisis Team

A Handbook for the Mental Health Professional

Medical Department
Harper & Row, Publishers
Hagerstown, Maryland
New York, Evanston, San Francisco, London

Standard Book Number: 06-141538-3

Library of Congress Catalog Card Number: 72-7758

For our wives Lynette Lieb and Susan Lipsitch, and our parents Benjamin and Rose Lieb, Lester and Miriam Lipsitch, and Andrew and Evelyn Slaby.

Contents

Preface   xi

Acknowledgements   xv

Foreword   xvii

Introduction   xix

THE STRUCTURE AND FUNCTION OF A CRISIS TEAM 1

A History of Crisis Intervention   3
The Crisis Intervention Unit   10
    The Director. The Head Nurse
The Crisis Team   15
    The Mental Health Professional
The Crisis Patient   22
The Unit's Relationship to the Community   27

THE PROCESS OF CRISIS INTERVENTION   31

The Intake   33
    Special Considerations Around Admission. The Pa-
    tient's Arrival on the Unit. Gathering Information
The Clinical Psychosocial Case History   40

The Mental Status Examination. The Medical Evaluation

Evaluation of Suicidal and Homicidal Potential   60
Evaluation of Suicide Risk. Evaluation of Homicidal Potential

Use of Psychotropic Agents   67
The Stay on the Crisis Unit   73
Disposition of Patients   77
The Evaluation of Patients for Referral. The Selection of Patients for Psychotherapy. Referrals Made From a Crisis Unit

**ILLUSTRATIVE EXAMPLES OF CRISIS
INTERVENTION**   87

The Psychotic Patient   89
The Manic Patient. The Acute Schizophrenic. The Chronic Schizophrenic. The Involutional Psychotic. The Patient with a Drug Psychosis
Patients for Detoxification   100
Drug Withdrawal. The Alcoholic for Detoxification
Crisis with Potential for Violence   104
The Domestic Crisis. The Homicidal Patient. The Suicidal Patient. The Melodrama. The Legal Referral
External Stress Crisis   114
The Acute Grief Reaction. The Transient Situational Crisis. The Therapy Crisis
Life Cycle Crisis   120
The Adolescent in Crisis. The Abortion Evaluation. The Postpartum Psychosis. The Geriatric Patient
Crisis of a Chronic Nature   130
The Resourceless Patient. The Resource-Devouring Patient. The Sociopathic Patient. The Character Disorder
The Diagnostic Puzzles   138
The Medical Case. A Diagnostic Puzzle. The Unusual Case

APPENDIXES 143

Psychosocial History Forms 145
    Noncomputerized Form. Computerized Form
Mental Status Forms 158
    Noncomputerized Form. Computerized Form
The Physical Examination Form 170

The Discharge Summary 172

REFERENCES 173

INDEX 179

Preface

"How are you able to get patients out so fast?" "Do you really mean you trust people without a medical background to take the history?" These questions are frequently asked by visitors from other communities. We hope this book answers these and other important questions raised by the concept of crisis intervention.

While numerous technical texts have been written on the phenomenology and psychodynamics of mental illness, most are intended for medical students and physicians. If there is to be a more egalitarian distribution of mental health services, much of the evaluation and care of patients will have to be entrusted to the important growing body of nonphysician mental health workers.

Both the Midtown (Srole *et al.*, 1962) and New Haven (Hollingshead and Redlich, 1958) studies focused attention on the prevalence of mental illness among the lower social classes. Moreover, the Midtown study shows that while the lower social classes have the greatest need, these people have the most difficulty in obtaining adequate psychiatric services.

In comprehensive terms, compared to the "affluent" groups the "poor" have many more mentally impaired people; their help-needy people far less often get psychiatric attention; and when their impaired members do get such attention, the outcome, to judge from an elicited clue, rather less often appears to be a significant and sustained gain.

The lack of available services to the indigent might well be due to the tendency of American psychiatry to place a high value on long-term intensive psychotherapy. However, even if shorter term therapies had

xi

been a common practice, not enough medically trained clinicians would have been available to provide service.

This gap is being closed by drawing mental health workers—professionals, as we call them in this book—from the ranks of nursing, social work, clergy, and the community itself, the latter often with no training beyond high school. These groups, especially that from the community, play an important role in the management of a crisis unit.

A multidisciplinary approach must be implemented by a multidisciplinary staff. While a psychiatrist may be called upon for diagnosis or consultation about the use of psychotropic drugs, a community mental health professional may provide what is equally valuable: an assessment of the patient's resources in the community and access to information about the patient. As clinicians, we see ourselves not only as psychotherapists, but as sociotherapists as well, moving from one pole to another depending on a patient's needs. A psychiatrist, often biased by his interest in psychopathology, may neglect the realities confronting a homeless, jobless, lower-class schizophrenic, while a worker less inculcated with psychodynamic theory may focus on factors more immediate to the patient's crisis, i.e., lack of structure on the most fundamental level—no job and no home.

Further, innovation and pragmatism are often lacking in traditional approaches which follow a particular theoretical model. Mental health professionals other than the psychiatrist can provide approaches which the psychiatrist would not dare to suggest because of his traditional theoretical orientation, but which he is happy to condone. In psychiatry there are no "right" answers but rather a variety of therapeutic approaches which can be chosen to suit a situation. Indeed, much of what has been accepted as dogma in psychiatry—and in medicine in general, such as the hospital treatment of some patients with heart attacks (Mathew *et al.*, 1971)—has never been put to the test empirically.

The mental health professional should be cognizant of the possibilities and limitations of psychiatry. We do not always cure, nor do we aim to. Some patients' intrapsychic difficulty or external reality situation is such that at most we can help them come to a compromise. As one of our patients wryly commented, "One cannot undo in five days what has been 25 years in the making." We realize this, but we try to bring about some positive change in the patient's life.

In an editorial in *The American Journal of Psychiatry* (March, 1972) David E. Raskin, M. D., of the National Institute of Mental Health commented, "I am thus suggesting . . . a willingness to share previously cherished areas of psychiatry with other mental health workers." In keeping with this spirit, it is our hope that the material presented here will be comprehensible and helpful to all members of a crisis team. Where possible we have tried to avoid burdensome jargon and to present our material so that the everyday functioning and tasks of a crisis unit can be understood by readers without previous psychiatric education. It is our opinion that enthusiasm, a sense of responsibility, empathy, native intelligence, and continuing proper training are the prerequisites for successful crisis work. We hope that this book will contribute substantially toward this training.

J.L.
I.I.L.
A.E.S.

Acknowledgements

The authors wish to express their gratitude to Boris M. Astrachan, Professor of Clinical Psychiatry, Yale University, and Jerome K. Myers, Professor of Sociology, Yale University, who contributed their suggestions, criticism, and support; to Arthur Frank, who proofread the manuscript; and to Jane Keane, who typed it. We also extend our gratitude to the members of the Crisis Intervention Unit at the Connecticut Mental Health Center whose challenging questions and innovative ideas prompted us to write this book.

Foreword

The crisis unit which served as a model for this book and from which the illustrative case examples have been drawn is a part of the Connecticut Mental Health Center, New Haven, Connecticut. The Center is the product of a collaboration between the Yale University Department of Psychiatry and the State of Connecticut. In participation with other community-based agencies, it provides comprehensive mental health services for the greater New Haven area. In addition to its defined primary task of clinical service, it is a major center for psychiatric research and training. Postdoctoral fellows in the Department of Psychiatry, graduate nursing students, and medical students at Yale join social work and psychology students from Smith College, Columbia University, Atlanta University and the University of Connecticut, community trainees, and students in other fields in integrated training programs.

Introduction

The remarkable development of crisis therapy as an accepted clinical intervention is signaled by the publication of this book. Having observed and participated in this development in the clinical facilities used by the Department of Psychiatry, Yale University School of Medicine, I was greatly pleased when asked to write this Introduction.

Crisis intervention training for residents in our department was limited to emergency room experience until the Connecticut Mental Health Center opened in 1966. At that time Dr. Claudewell Thomas developed an Emergency Treatment Service which provided brief hospital treatment and 30-day outpatient follow-up for individuals in acute distress. During its first few years this service was utilized only rarely as a training placement for residents since its training resources were initially committed to the education of the staff that provided direct service.

The effectiveness of this Emergency Treatment Service, and its acceptance by patients, professionals, and the community, eventuated in significant reallocation of institutional resources to this form of treatment. Psychiatric residents, students of social work, nursing and psychology, and allied health worker trainees become involved in this work, enabling trainees with a variety of clinical and theoretical backgrounds to work together effectively. Presently, acute intervention experience within a variety of hospital and community settings has become a required part of the training program for residents in the Yale Department of Psychiatry.

Due to increased utilization of crisis therapy, critical questions are raised about current standards of ethical practice in crisis intervention.

Standards and practices of confidentiality and privacy must be reassessed as the family is involved in treatment. By shifting the clinical focus from the isolated patient to the patient within the context of family and other social systems the long established responsibility of therapist to patient is modified. The clinician acts as agent not of the patient but of the patient and family. The patient's thoughts, wishes and behavior are considered along with those of family members, friends, etc. Obviously, the privacy of the patient is accorded less weight than the work of treatment, so confidentiality is guaranteed the family, not the individual.

The therapist acts from a position of relative power. Because of his expertise, societally ascribed status and interest in the patient's functioning, his opinion is accorded weight. He is not a disinterested neutral observer. His judgements, hopefully made in careful consultation with all the parties involved, are governed by his concern for improved interpersonal functioning and diminished intrapsychic distress.

We may anticipate that treatment settings which provide crisis intervention will develop evaluative procedures to continually monitor not only the appropriateness and the quality of care, but also the ethical standards under which care is delivered. This concern with ethics must inevitably involve an informed public in the direct review of patient care.

Crisis intervention extends the scope of the clinical activities of mental health professionals. The interdisciplinary staff necessary to the functioning of crisis units not only provides rich training resources for teaching the techniques of crisis intervention, but also for collaboratively exploring issues of therapist activity, values and problems of confidentiality and privacy.

Boris M. Astrachan, M.D.
Professor of Clinical Psychiatry, Yale University School of Medicine; Director, Connecticut Mental Health Center, New Haven, Connecticut

The Crisis Team

THE STRUCTURE AND
FUNCTION OF A CRISIS TEAM

A History of Crisis Intervention

Crisis intervention has adapted to constantly changing demands placed upon it by conditions in various communities. Much of what is practiced on crisis units today would seem alien to early theorists in the field as it is the result of developments that began with psychiatrists' experiences during World War II and have evolved through recent critical evaluations of long-term therapies. These evaluations have suggested that the economics of an equitable distribution of mental health services make the use of longer-term therapies infeasible. The factors which have contributed to the development of crisis intervention technique are:

1. The experience gained from treating combat emergencies during wartime
2. The discovery of certain "generic" (Jacobson, 1968) patterns of response to various crisis situations confronting "normal" individuals
3. The construction of a theoretical model of the psychodynamics of life crises and their resolution
4. The demand for a range of mental health services appropriate to the needs of all socioeconomic classes
5. An increased understanding of the detrimental effects of longer-term psychiatric hospitalization such as institutionalism (Goffman, 1961)
6. The evolution of brief or emergency psychotherapeutic techniques, both on an inpatient and outpatient basis

3

7. Evaluative studies suggesting that briefer hospitalization may be as efficacious—or better in some situations—than the traditional longer-term hospitalization (Weisman *et al.*, 1969).

Experience derived from treating soldiers during the last three major wars indicates that in order to prevent regression and the development of more entrenched patterns of psychiatric illness, an early return to combat units is important (Glass, 1954; Hausman and Rioch, 1967; Menninger, 1948). It is apparent from physicians treating soldiers during war that persisting dysfunction is reduced by using supportive psychotherapeutic techniques at treatment centers as near to the front lines as possible. The patient's knowledge that he has to return to combat counters his regressive tendencies and prevents him and others from labeling him a psychiatric casualty—a role he would frequently want to assume because of its obvious secondary gain. Unfortunately, such a role generally leads to greater regression and more permanent maladaptive patterns of behavior. The factors outlined by Caldwell (1967), such as locating treatment facilities as far forward in combat zones as possible, focusing on the immediate situational crisis and an individual's feelings about what has happened to him, promotion of group support, social manipulation, adequate rest, and rapid return to combat duties in an effort to maintain self-confidence in his own ability to function, can be applied to the treatment of patients in community-based crisis centers. With minimum interference in a person's life routine, and with commitment to returning him or her to functioning in his own milieu, regression is undercut; like the soldiers in acute crises who could function as well as other troops once they returned to duty, it has been found that patients treated similarly can be returned to their families, friends, and work.

The second major contribution to the development of current concepts of crisis intervention originated in 1944 with Lindemann's classic study on the symptomatology and management of acute grief reactions. Referred to by Jacobson *et al.* (1968) as the "generic" approach, it emphasizes the definition of characteristic behavior patterns which seem to develop in response to particular life crises. Treatment programs based on an understanding of these patterns deemphasize the variation in individual psychodynamics. Lindemann (1944), for example, discusses the course of bereavement seen in relatives of those who died in the catastrophic Coconut Grove fire. Studies have also been done of patterns of response to a premature birth (Kaplan and Mason,

1960; Caplan, 1964), the diagnosis of chronicity and impending surgery (Janis, 1958), and points in the course of marital life which are vulnerable to unusual stresses (Rapoport, 1963).

While studies such as Lindemann's deal with situations seldom encountered in either community or private psychiatric practice, they do provide models for programs of primary prevention based on adaptive resolution of the crisis situation. Unfortunately, these models are not appropriate for a crisis unit, where most of the treatment is of a secondary preventative nature and more akin to the treatment of combat reactions, e.g., reintegrating a schizophrenic, providing brief supportive therapy for a patient undergoing a grief reaction.

An outcome of the increased knowledge of the patterns of response to life crises has been the attempt to develop a theoretical framework which would lead to a better understanding of the intrapsychic changes that correlate with the overt responses to a crisis (Caplan, 1959, 1961, 1964; Thomas and Weisman, 1951; Porter, 1966; Parad and Caplan, 1965; Rapoport, 1965; and Darbonne, 1968). A theory of acute emotional disorder, as noted by Kaplan and Mason (1960), has been developed from understanding the so-called traumatic neuroses (Freud, 1925; Kardiner, 1941; Fenichel, 1945) and from an understanding of acute infectious diseases (Halliday, 1943) as well as from the work on acute grief reactions. The course of such a disorder is thought to be limited usually to four to six weeks with a median of about four weeks (Jacobson, 1965). While not denying that the underlying intrapsychic organization may make some people more susceptible to disintegration (e.g., early loss of parents increasing one's vulnerability to the stress of a later loss of a love object), such a theory generally emphasizes the extrapsychic realities which may in fact be overtaxing a well-balanced person. This emphasis has often distinguished clinicians doing crisis work from more traditional-oriented psychotherapists. The emotional discord and unhappiness experienced by individuals at times of stress, such as divorce and separation, rather than being viewed as indicants of psychopathology are viewed by the crisis clinician as responses that can be understood—and treated, if indicated—without refering to early psychogenetic experiences. These situations can be seen in much the same perspective as Erikson's (1950) concept of developmental crisis as a time for growth. Successful mastery of a crisis will often equip an individual to cope with future crises in a more mature way. Emphasis is placed on the recruitment of community and other social supports which may complement intrapsychic ego function at a time when the equilibrium between external reality factors and intrapsychic organization is disturbed. Caplan (1964) succinctly describes a crisis as

A short period of psychological disequilibrium in a person who confronts a hazardous circumstance that for him constitutes an important problem which he can for the time being neither escape nor solve with his customary problem-solving resources.

During the period of upset when a person's intrapsychic defenses are inadequate, he is vulnerable to external forces, be they malevolent forces in his own environment or the forces that exist in the hospital. Because of this increased plasticity, a little effort appropriately applied can often shift the balance from mental illness to mental health. This is consistent with the preventive psychiatric orientation of crisis work (Caplan, 1961–1962).

Long-lasting results depend on the availability of psychosocial supports; therefore, emphasis in crisis work should be placed on assessing the immediate environmental props, be they the patient's family, lover, employer, or local community groups such as the church, etc. The structure of the patient's family, the interaction between family members, the patient's social role and his social network should be assessed (Parad, 1965). The concept that one's environment comprises a matrix which complements his own intrapsychic defenses at times of crisis has been discussed by Lindemann (1953) and the Leightons (1959, 1963).

Psychiatry has been remiss in providing mental health services for the lower socioeconomic classes and for older people. These people frequently fail to get accepted into outpatient treatment programs, and when they do, they often get little more than a diagnostic work-up (Brill and Storrow, 1960; Hollingshead and Redlich, 1958; Hunt, 1960; Jacobson, 1965; Lief *et al.*, 1961; Reusch, 1953;). The problem is compounded because such people do not usually respond well to classic psychiatric approaches such as psychoanalytic psychotherapy. Psychiatrists trained in the traditional manner are sometimes unable to respond to what these patients are really seeking when they consult a therapist, and the dissimilarity in backgrounds serves to further alienate the patient. It is, therefore, no surprise when these patients fail to follow through in outpatient treatment.

During the 1950s, concomitant with an increased awareness of the inequitable distribution of mental health services was a growing cognizance of the detrimental effects of long-term hospitalization. Goffman (1961) and others (Stanton and Schwartz, 1954; Wing, 1967) have discussed phenomena such as institutionalism and deculturation and have defined characteristics of a social breakdown syndrome that results from a variety of factors operant in "total" institutions such as the large state mental hospitals. Individuals appear to abandon their executive ego functions as they increasingly assume a compliant role in a social system in which nearly all rewards for their operant behavior, be they physical, psychological, or social, are contingent on their adherence to a behavior pattern deemed appropriate by the administrative staff. That this phenomenon is not restricted to large, understaffed state hospitals but may also be found in richly endowed private institutions, where more in-depth therapy is practiced, has been suggested by Feirstein *et al.* (1971), who believe that such a setting encourages a patient to envision his difficulty as the result of a lifelong development of maladaptive patterns of response. While this may indeed be true, the tacit message is that in order to deal with the present dysfunction long-term treatment is necessary. But this leaves the many patients who are unable both financially and psychologically to utilize such a treatment program only too ready to assume the role of the psychiatric casualty.

The evolution of crisis theory, the desire for a better distribution of mental health services, and the desire to discourage the regression and deculturation seen in longer-term hospitals have lead to the technique of brief or emergency treatments. While there are obvious logistic differences between brief techniques when applied to outpatients as opposed to inpatient units, there are certain characteristics which distinguish them from the traditional longer psychotherapeutic techniques. This has been discussed by Aquilera (1970), Bellak and Small (1965), Feirstein *et al.* (1971), Jacobson *et al.* (1968), and Thomas and Weisman (1970) and can be briefly outlined as follows:

1. Treatment contracts are time-limited. This is important for the patient and his family. The patient develops a set that he has only a limited time in which to resolve his difficulty and return to his own milieu. At the same time, the patient's family and friends do not begin to identify him as a hopeless psychiatric casualty.

2. Psychotropic agents are freely employed for symptomatic relief. Medication is liberally used to alleviate ego-alien symptoms and facilitate rapid return to premorbid levels of functioning. Being able to maintain role performance—and to obtain the needed sleep and anxiety-reduction to effect this—is seen as an integral part of brief treatment. It is unrealistic to assume that major psychodynamic changes can occur in time-limited therapy.

3. Active use of the relevant social systems. The therapist pragmatically involves others in order to return the patient to his usual level of functioning. This may include not only family members but also

friends, employers, and clergy. If the return of the patient to functioning requires active environmental manipulation, this is promptly effected. Families, for example, are more susceptible to manipulation in times of crisis than at times when there is less tension and anxiety.

4. Patients may be seen by more than one therapist. That which is deemed anathema to most conventional therapies is routine on some crisis units. The advantage in treatment which discourages regression and dependence is obvious. The patient can remain more autonomous and is supported, as on the outside, by many others. There is not the over-dependence on the somewhat deified person of "the doctor," to whom a patient may wish to abandon all sense of autonomy in times of crisis.

5. The focus is on the current life situation. Again, if one is to return a patient quickly to his environment, an understanding of factors immediately impeding his return is essential. This is not to devalue the longitudinal history for diagnostic and prognostic purposes, but rather to place emphasis on the current life situation.

6. Multiple therapies are employed during a treatment course. This applies more to inpatient than outpatient treatment. Individual, group, family, and couples therapy may be used at the same time for both assessment and therapeutic purposes. Psychodrama, sodium amytal interviews, and other techniques may also be employed.

7. A positive attitude towards the staff is encouraged. Care, understanding, and competence usually generate a sense of trust. A feeling that the person has support and can be helped is important in facilitating rapid discharge.

8. Staff is drawn from several social, educational, age and ethnic backgrounds. This enables a patient to feel that there are those about him who can empathize with his needs. It also provides a variety of people who may contribute to the planning of treatment programs for patients from a particular ethnic subculture.

9. The emphasis placed on verbalizing one's intrapsychic strife is less than in long-term psychotherapies. The inability of a patient to relate in a meaningful way what is bothering him and to identify what he sees as the precipitants of his crisis is not deemed a contraindication to treatment the way it might be in longer insight-oriented psychotherapies.

10. An attempt is made to restore the patient's self-esteem and self-

reliance. The relationship between the therapist, or therapists, and the patient is quite different to that seen in more traditional psychotherapies. Patient and therapist often collaborate in deciding on the need for and nature of follow-up treatment, including in some instances the continuance of hospitalization.

Studies of innovative approaches to the treatment of grossly psychotic patients have been illuminating. Pasamanick's (1967) study indicated that schizophrenics treated at home may do as well as those hospitalized. An earlier study by Weisman *et al.* (1967) of an emergency treatment facility where the stay was limited to three to five days indicated that the rehospitalization or transfer rate after two years did not differ remarkably from that found in studies of hospitals comparably staffed, with average patient stays of three weeks, four months, and eight months (Friedman *et al.*, 1966: Levenstein *et al.*, 1966; Wilder *et al.*, 1966). This has remarkable implications given the fact that the patient population included 38% diagnosed as psychotic and 10% as borderline psychotic. The concept that rehospitalization comprises a treatment failure is undergoing scrutiny. Readmission rates have been rising since 1953 (U.S.P.H.S., 1963) and will probably remain at the current or higher levels as we become increasingly adept at keeping patients out of state hospitals through the use of episodic brief hospitalizations in community-based centers.

The Crisis Intervention Unit

While the structure of crisis units may vary, the essential personnel are a unit director, a head nurse, and the members of the team or teams. The fundamental working unit and the most important constituent of crisis intervention is the team. For this reason the next chapter is devoted entirely to a discussion of the team. In addition to the director, the unit may need to employ one or two psychiatrists to act as his assistants, especially on units where there is a rapid turnover of many patients.

THE DIRECTOR

The director should be a psychiatrist, preferably one who has broad experience in clinical psychiatry, psychodynamics, psychopharmacology, and social psychiatry. It is important for the director to be interested in and believe in the efficacy of crisis work and in the ability of nonpsychiatric professionals to act as primary clinicians. It is an advantage for him or her to be a psychiatrist—or at least a psychiatrically oriented physician—for the following reasons:

1. Medicolegal Considerations. Whenever drugs are prescribed on an inpatient unit and when factors such as suicide and homicide come into play, the ultimate responsibility for patient care resides with a physician.
2. Medical Illness. Patients with acute medical illnesses such as acute

intoxication, and chronic medical illnesses such as diabetes, often present on a crisis unit. Early diagnosis and prompt institution of the appropriate treatment, or a request for consultation, are mandatory. As it is the director's task to coordinate the treatment of every patient admitted, it is best if he has a medical and psychiatric background so that rapid distinction can be made between cases that require medical attention and those that do not.

3. Neuropsychiatric evaluation and the use of psychotropic medications are key factors in successful crisis work.

4. The director must be perceived by the unit and by the institution as a competent clinician and administrator who can muster up resources for the optimal running of the unit. It is also valuable if he is seen as a person who can deal effectively with outside agencies as well as with other units within the institution—inpatient units, outpatient departments, or an evaluation service.

5. Often patients and their families will symbolize physicians as people who heal. Social workers, senior nurses, and aides, however competent, are given symbolic representations by the public and by staff members. Situations arise on a crisis unit where a recalcitrant patient or an obstinate family will ask for a meeting with the "doctor" and will often defer to his judgement and accept his recommendations.

FUNCTIONS OF THE DIRECTOR

Although the functions of the director would vary from unit to unit, there are certain tasks that might be considered basic:

1. The director oversees the crisis management of every admission and strives for a high standard of care for each case.

2. The director stays informed of the clinical problems presented by each patient and advises team members on questions relating to diagnosis, medication, outside consultations, therapeutic interviews, and disposition.

3. The director, with the head nurse, coordinates staff duties: assignment of staff members to a particular team, equitable distribution of work (particularly weekend duties), and supervision of staff members. The supervision of the clinicians on a crisis unit serves a number of purposes as follows:

a. Clinical. Individual staff members can discuss issues pertaining to the management of their current case load, both inpatient and outpatient.

b. Teaching.   Topics such as interviewing skills, diagnosis and treatment of mental disorders, and the use of community agencies can be covered.

c. Administration.   Problems arising from the processing of discharge or transfer summaries and the effecting of referrals can be dealt with.

d. Special consideration.   Crisis work is at times taxing and can be unrewarding when a series of difficult or intractable cases present within a short space of time. Therefore, it is important for the supervisors to be sensitive to morale and to be aware of how staff members are faring in their clinical responsibilities from week to week.

4. Finally, the director can provide through his personality and ability a model of a competent crisis clinician. In this regard it is instructive and morale boosting when the director from time to time assigns himself as primary clinician to a patient and personally performs all the clinical and administrative tasks inherent in this role.

THE HEAD NURSE

The head nurse plays an important role in the immediate organization of the unit. She assigns the psychiatric nurses, aides, and trainees to the teams and arranges their rotation through the day, evening, and night shifts. Together with the director, she supervises patient care and alerts clinicians to the needs of their patients.

For effective crisis work to occur, there should exist a strong esprit de corps and sense of professional responsibility. Intra and interteam strife has to be kept to a minimum, and it is the head nurse's task to attempt to work out difficulties when they occur. It is the head nurse's responsibility to function both as an intermediary between the nursing staff and the physicians and as the representative of the nursing staff within the total institution. She is a figure around whom much role modeling should occur and should therefore set a high standard both in terms of her personal demeanor and behavior and in her work with the staff and the patients, in order to be respected, trusted, and liked. It is incumbent on the head nurse, like the director, to know her staff well and to be readily available to them for consultation.

The nature of crisis work demands that the unit be designed to admit patients at all times and that treatment be started as soon as a patient is admitted. For this reason, the crisis unit operates seven days a week without any decrease in admissions or discharges on weekends. Since patients may need to stay for only a day or two, it is not uncommon for a patient admitted on Saturday to be discharged the next day.

Although the design of a crisis unit may differ from place to place, there are certain principles that should be adhered to. To begin with, a reasonable amount of structure should be built into each day. As with any inpatient unit, it is helpful to both staff and patients if there is a certain routine to follow. For each patient the day should be arranged so that a certain number of hours are spent in individual interviews, family meetings, or other planned therapeutic activities. Sufficient time must be set aside, however, to allow patients to pursue activities geared towards discharge, e.g. job hunting, visits home, and appointments with outpatient therapists. For the staff, forums must exist where members can share information, discuss new admissions, plan for discharges, and seek advice from one another or from the director and his assistants.

On the Crisis Intervention Unit at the Connecticut Mental Health Center the staff as a whole meets for an hour every afternoon to discuss all the patients on the unit. This forum, which is termed "rounds", serves the following functions:

1. Staff members exchange ideas and share expertise.
2. The unit director uses the information provided to make suggestions pertaining to diagnosis and management
3. The transfer of responsibility to evening staff is effected. A treatment focus for each patient is suggested to the evening staff by the clinicians who have been involved with patients during the day.
4. New and expected admissions are presented.
5. A forum is provided for the director and his assistants to use the case material presented to highlight important aspects of psychodynamics, psychopathology, and therapeutic technique.

The following is a format of a day's activities on the Crisis Intervention Unit at the Connecticut Mental Health Center. It has proved effective for this unit, but this is not to say that it could not be substantially altered.

8:00 A.M.	Breakfast
8:15 A.M.	Blood drawing
8:30 A.M.	Team meeting: staff discussion group
8:45 A.M.	Team meeting: assessment and planning group (with patients)
9:30 A.M.	Team meeting: staff wrap-up

10:00 A.M.	Interviews with patients and family members, information gathering from other sources
12:00 noon	Lunch
1:00 P.M.	Interviews with patients and family members, information gathering from other sources
3:00 P.M.	Rounds
4:00 P.M.	Interviews with patients and family members, information gathering
5:00 P.M.	Dinner
5:30 P.M.	Interviews with patients and family members, information gathering
8:30 P.M.	Evening group (one hour)
10:00 P.M.	Patients retire

The task of the evening staff is to interview family members, clarify important issues with patients and run a group therapy session. The patients on the unit are encouraged to ventilate their feelings about the day in a relatively informal setting, to share experiences and provide each other with support, and to make practical suggestions geared toward discharge.

The evening and night staff accept new admissions at any hour from referring clinicians. Patients admitted during the evening and night receive an intensive work-up which is passed on to the staff coming on duty in the morning.

The director, his assistants and the head nurse provide rotational back-up coverage to the unit and can be contacted at any time by the staff.

Patients generally spend most of the day on the unit, but if they are deemed well enough they are allowed out on pass to purchase food, cigarettes, etc., or to go to work or to school.

Visiting hours are in the afternoon and evening, and the unit is generally open unless there is a highly psychotic patient who, in his confusion or desire to test limits, might try to leave. However, the door is seldom kept locked for more than a day as we feel that this encourages regression and acting out behavior among patients and diminishes staff morale. The open door represents a symbolic and real continuity with the outside world to which the patients must quickly return. It is for this reason that the location of crisis units on the first floor of an institution is especially appropriate.

The Crisis Team

The fundamental unit of crisis intervention service is the team. The team consists of four to six clinicians of various professional identifications and levels of training. In our setting there are one or two nurses, a psychiatric aide, a social worker, and a psychiatrist. In addition, there are trainees from various disciplines who join the team during their rotations through the crisis unit and are assigned either full or partial responsibility for patient care depending on their competence, level of industry, and sense of responsibility. This means that in addition to the core of four to six team members there will be at any one time four to six additional members drawn from the medical school, social work school, divinity school, and the community.

Individual team members function for a few weeks at a time as the "group leader." It is this person's duty to run the morning meeting, coordinate staff's activities during the day, and to present the patients' progress to rounds in the afternoon.

Each morning the crisis team meets as a group. A succinct report is made on each patient's progress since the previous afternoon and newly admitted patients are briefly presented and discussed. The reports consist mostly of abstracts of the notes in the patients' charts.

Following the conclusion of the reports, the patients are brought into the morning meeting. There is an initial introduction of patients and staff to each other, and then the group leader initiates a brief interview with each patient. Other staff members involve themselves in this task as well. Patients are not encouraged to interact with each other but are not prevented from doing so if they choose and if it seems helpful. At the end of his interview, the patient is asked what issues he would like to work on during the day and is told that a staff member will be talking to him later in the morning.

Next the staff meets to discuss the patients and plan the day. The group leader coordinates the discussion on each patient and takes notes on what will be the focus for each patient during the day. When this meeting ends, staff members leave to pursue their tasks; during the day the group leader assimilates information pertinent to the patients' progress and records this in his notes.

At afternoon rounds each team is presented separately to the entire staff on the unit. Each group leader coordinates the presentation of each patient on the team and calls upon the staff members to present their patients' progress. There is a free interchange of ideas between the staff members, and decisions are made on each patient pertaining to a focus for the evening staff to follow. Discharge will frequently be a topic, and in that case, much time is accorded to planning for it. New and expected admissions are briefly presented and changes in unit policy, general issues, and staff suggestions are aired.

When a patient arrives on the unit, he is assigned a primary clinician. A staff member usually volunteers for this role and individual preferences are respected. If a staff member is interested in a particular individual, and if he feels he can quickly establish a therapeutic relationship, so much the better. The primary clinician bears the primary responsibility for the patient's care, starting with the evaluation and ending with the discharge summary. From time to time other staff members will fill in (e.g., when the primary clinician has the day off, or on weekends). When a complicated situation arises, specialized intervention may be requested, e.g., the involvement of a social worker with a difficult family. The primary clinician is expected to be aware of any changes in the patient's situation and is the clinician with whom the family, referring psychiatrists, and outside agencies will negotiate. He is also responsible for arranging follow-up care and for staying in touch with the patient until the referral has been effected. Occasionally, it is appropriate for the primary clinician to himself provide a 30-day follow-up program for his patient.

Three principles are key to an understanding of how the team functions on the crisis unit now in operation at the Connecticut Mental Health Center. First is the interchangeability of roles. One of the unique characteristics of the team is built-in continuity of patient care. While each team member's special qualifications or talents are recognized and used when possible, any member may interview the patient, relative, or a friend. Phone calls to previous therapists or school counselors, or obtaining a patient's previous records are also tasks which may be performed by any member of the team. Thus, various aspects of a patient's treatment can be undertaken concurrently. While a nurse is interviewing the patient, an aide may be talking to the parents, and a psychiatrist may be consulting with the family physician. These roles, or tasks, might be easily interchanged.

Second, the decisions involving the patient are group decisions. There are few unilateral decisions on the crisis unit, and most decisions are made by consensus, usually during rounds but also during informal discussion between staff members who have been involved with a patient. Often, the psychiatrist will outline what is clinically indicated for the patient, and thereafter the implementation of the plan and decisions around it, e.g., time of discharge and outpatient follow-up, are made by team members. It is one of the tasks of the psychiatrist to observe the decision-making and to ensure that the staff members' personal feelings do not become a major issue around the treatment of a particular patient; e.g., attractive adolescents often ruffle the feathers of female nursing staff with the result being a push for premature discharge.

Third is task orientation. From the time of arrival to the time of discharge the staff has to clearly keep in mind what the goals of the patient's treatment are. The moment it is clear that the goals have been achieved—or that they are highly unlikely to be achieved—the patient is discharged. It is not infrequent for a patient to be discharged on the same day that he is admitted. It is essential for all to keep in mind the reason for the patient's admission. There are, unfortunately but unavoidably, times when certain persons might have a special interest in imposing unrealistic expectations on the unit in terms of "my patient" or "my husband." At times like this it is important that everyone on the unit understands what the issues are so that excessive conflict does not arise around management of the patient.

The following descriptions relate to the unique task responsibilities of the various members of the crisis teams at the Connecticut Mental Health Center:

1. Nurses. The nurses on the crisis teams function like the other team members, but in addition they are responsible for providing medication for the patients and performing other nursing functions, e.g., taking vital signs when necessary. Charting, however, is not a specific nursing function but is done by all the team members. The

psychiatric nurse, because of her training and experience, is often the most alert to changes in the patient's social interactions, general behavior, and eating and sleeping patterns.

2. Psychiatric Aides and Community Workers. These individuals are drawn from varying backgrounds and a wide range of disciplines, e.g., religion, psychology, and education. They frequently have intimate knowledge about the life styles and stress that the patients are exposed to, and the resources in the community. Often they can establish a unique rapport with patients from a particular socioeconomic or ethnic stratum and thus become essential to the effective functioning of the team.

3. The Psychiatrist. The psychiatrist oversees the treatment of all the patients on his team. Generally, it is best for the psychiatrist to take a back seat. He does, however, attend all the morning meetings and the rounds to add his observations to the evaluations and decision making and to intervene in especially difficult situations. He is available all day to consult with team members about clinical and administrative issues. It is is important that even when he is not directly involved in the management of a patient, he is visible to patients and staff during the day as an integrating force on a unit, which by definition is somewhat unstructured. The psychiatrist is of particular value to the team with respect to questions of diagnosis, medication, and administrative issues such as the number of new admissions that can be taken during a period when the unit is already carrying a number of very disturbed patients. He is available throughout the day, and on a nightly telephone rotation, to supervise staff both on inpatient and outpatient problems.

4. Social Workers. Social workers carry out much the same function as other team members but provide in addition special expertise in family evaluation and outside agency referrals.

5. Students. The team approach provides a unique opportunity for supervised inpatient training in crisis work. Medical students, divinity students, social work students, graduate nursing students, and students from community mental health programs are encouraged to function as primary clinicians and to participate in the total functioning of the unit. Because of the interchangeability of roles, the emphasis on group decision, and the team approach, students are allowed to assume tasks commensurate with their maturity, their sense of responsibility, and their skills.

6. The Clergy. A chaplain or a divinity student is often a valuable member of a crisis team. For many middle-and lower-class patients

the clergy play an important role in the community. Divinity students are frequently aware of facilities that churches have for persons without resources. We have had patients whose main source of social contact had been church groups, and the reestablishing of these contacts proved valuable in their discharge planning.

THE MENTAL HEALTH PROFESSIONAL

People electing to work in the mental health field are most effective when they possess certain personal attributes together with the ability to assume the professional characteristics necessary when working with acutely disturbed individuals. Characteristics that contribute to the making of a mature, competent clinician include an interest in the vagaries of human nature, warmth, empathy, and the ability to accept deviance and tolerate ambiguity.

When beginning this book we debated whether to call it A Handbook for Mental Health *Workers* or Mental Health *Professionals.* We decided on the latter because we felt that there are characteristics that distinguish a "professional" from a "worker," and it is the professional qualities which make an individual, regardless of his training, able to assume the role of a primary clinician on a crisis unit. The characteristics we deem important for professionals are:

1. A Sense of Responsibility. While this may seem obvious, it is the characteristic least displayed by those who prefer to work on a more traditional psychiatric unit where there is an authoritarian ward structure in which the psychiatrist assumes the responsibility. The responsibilities of a crisis worker may range from integrating all the information gathered on a patient to organizing his treatment on the unit and ultimately arranging for his follow-up care following discharge.

2. The Ability to Tolerate Anxiety. Working with psychiatric patients can often be anxiety-producing both because of the responsibilities for care involved and because of the subjective experiences aroused by working with particular kinds of patients. Strong reactions to particular patients are often natural, but it takes maturity to recognize these feelings so that they do not interfere in working with such patients. Suicidal and homicidal patients invariably provoke anxiety in those who work with them. The anxiety is inevitable, but it is important that it not be allowed to interfere with rational decisions. Decision making, particularly when radical

changes in a patient's life may be effected, always causes anxiety. Due to the unstructured nature of a crisis unit and the urgency to make decisions, tension usually exists which can be handled only if the clinician is mature and can tolerate uncertainty and ambiguity.

3. The Ability to Handle One's Feelings. Feelings of anger, warmth, pity, disgust, embarrassment, guilt, and at times sexual feelings will be aroused in clinicians by their patients. Again, there is nothing wrong in experiencing them if they remain within acceptable limits, are not expressed to the patient, and do not interfere with treatment.

4. Appropriateness of Behavior. As a professional in the community, the clinician must be careful not to engage in behavior which in any way might be harmful to a patient or his family. A professional relationship with a patient includes his family. All contacts with a patient or his family should be limited to a helping capacity undertaken only on the unit.

   As a consequence of the therapeutic relationship, no matter how brief, the patient often develops warm feelings towards the clinician. For some patients the therapeutic relationship may allow a degree of intimacy never experienced before. The patient in a crisis situation may reveal things about himself to his clinician because he feels upset and helpless. This interaction may make him feel close and accepted, and often he would like to keep all or part of that experience. He might see his clinician as a savior, a good father, or a strong protector. These ideas comprise an exaggeration based on the patient's own relative state of helplessness as well as his need to see the person who helps him as very strong. If these distortions are kept in mind, any relationship outside the hospital cannot help but be somewhat unrealistic and in the long run will be harmful to the patient, his family, or the clinician himself.

5. The Ability to Maintain Confidentiality. It is not unusual for a staff member on a crisis unit to already know a patient. In fact, as mentioned previously, this staff member can provide useful information about the circumstances in which the patient and his family live. However, none of the highly personal information that a patient may reveal, or even the fact that he is on the unit, is discussible off the unit. Information pertaining to a clinician's dealings with patients and family members should be discussed only within the confines of the unit, a restriction that must be rigidly adhered to in order to ensure good care.

6. The Ability to Work on a Team. It often appeals to a novice to

monopolize a patient so that he will see him as *the* clinician to the exclusion of all others. With emphasis on the interchangeability of roles and a team approach, information must be freely shared and special relationships with patients avoided.

The team structure on a crisis unit demands free exchange of information and a working together for the patient's good. Team members have to help each other out in difficult situations, confer with each other about decisions, and share responsibility for the total care of patients.

7. The Ability to Work With Community Agencies. Involvement of other agencies, clinicians, or specialists in a particular field is often indicated in crisis work. Tapping these resources is frequently the responsibility of the clinician, and it is essential that he be able to establish rapport with useful outsiders.

The Crisis Patient

Attempting an exact definition of *crisis patient* can lead one into a maze of theoretical constructs. The definition we propose is a pragmatic one which, while not in line with some of the classical concepts of crisis discussed by Parad (1965) or Lindemann (1944), has enabled us to develop an approach which applies to the patients we see. Webster's Dictionary (1964) defines a crisis as

1. The turning point in the course of a disease, when it becomes clear whether the patient will recover or die. 2. A turning point in the course of anything; decisive or crucial time, stage, or event. 3. A crucial situation; situation whose outcome decides whether possible bad consequences will follow; as, an economic crisis. - Syn., see emergency.

While death is generally not a question in crisis patients save perhaps some suicidal ones, they are at a turning point. The adaptive mechanisms which have established their equilibrium and have sufficed before are either inadequate or inappropriate for the stress they face. The patient experiences a helplessness which is often shared by his friends and relatives. When he presents himself for help, either he feels unable to take action to solve his problem, or the actions he proposes are destructive to himself or others.

Aquilera *et al.* (1970) point out that crisis intervention offers the patient immediate help in reestablishing his equilibrium by providing inexpensive short-term treatment. Traditionally, this has involved the treatment of people with clearly defined environmental stresses such as the loss of a job, death in the family, or a marital difficulty. We propose expanding this to include people with clearly defined *intra-*

psychic crises. Thus we are able to include those patients who are undergoing their first psychotic break or the recurrence of long-standing quiescent psychotic symptoms. While these patients have not been officially included in the concept of crisis intervention, we have found that as mental health professionals have become more skilled in handling problems such as bereavement and suicidal gestures on an outpatient basis, more patients who have in the past been referred to a long-term hospital have been referred to the crisis unit. Sometimes this is for evaluation, but other times it is at the request of relatives who want an opportunity to work with the staff in helping to get the patient out of the hospital as soon as possible. Some of the patients might be unable to recompensate in the few days allotted on the crisis unit, but we are willing to try and have been impressed with our results. We do not aim so much to "cure" as to comfort, and to enable the patient to return to his family or other social setting with some gains having been made.

The types of patient we encounter fall into nine general groupings:

1. Patients with traditional crisis situations, e.g., acute bereavement, marital discord, suicidal gestures.
2. Patients with acute toxic reactions to drugs, e.g., L.S.D. trips, acute alcoholic intoxication.
3. Patients who are destructive to themselves or to others; e.g., severely depressed patients who wish to kill themselves, explosive personalities who want to or have injured others.
4. Patients with acute psychotic reactions, e.g., acute schizophrenic breaks, manic reactions. In this context it is important to note that the manics we have seen have frequently failed to respond and have had to be transferred to longer-term wards.
5. Patients who are chronically psychotic who present with an acute exacerbation, e.g., schizophrenics who have discontinued their medication or have experienced a severe stress such as a loss in the family.
6. Patients who are addicted to drugs or alcohol and are admitted for withdrawal.
7. Patients with questionable organic pathology who are unable to be managed on the outside; e.g., senile dementia, encephalitis.
8. Pregnant patients, generally adolescents, who are admitted for evaluation for an abortion.
9. Patients with a variety of other problems which are rarely seen today; e.g., fugue states, conversion reactions.

It is our policy to accept virtually all referrals, with the exception of dangerously assaultive, chronically regressed or heavily intoxicated patients. The management of these patients usually requires a locked door and constant staff attention which compromises the treatment of the other patients. Moreover, these patients do not generally respond to acute time-limited intervention.

SOURCES OF REFERRAL

The sources of referral to a crisis unit are multiple, but can be subdivided into two main categories.

Clinicians Who Effect Admissions to the Unit

These persons are distinguished both by their ability to perform a thorough psychiatric evaluation and by their understanding of the functioning of the crisis unit, its tasks, and its goals. This category includes:

1. Psychiatrists in general psychiatric practices
2. Psychoanalysts and psychotherapists
3. Psychiatrists working in emergency rooms
4. Psychiatric consultants to general medical and surgical services
5. Therapists in the outpatient psychiatric departments of general hospitals, mental health centers, and other psychiatric institutions
6. Clinicians who work in the psychiatric evaluation units of general hospitals, mental health centers, and other psychiatric institutions
7. Clinicians associated with various treatment programs, such as drug dependency units and alcohol clinics.

Individuals Who Initiate Admissions to the Unit

These persons are generally responsible for bringing patients to the attention of the individuals listed above. Anyone in the community can and often does function in this capacity, but the most common sources include:

1. Family members or friends
2. Family doctors
3. The police or lawyers
4. Health maintenance organizations
5. Family service organizations
6. Churches

7. Schools and colleges (especially student health services)
8. The patient himself

What distinguishes these individuals is that they are usually the first to perceive that something is amiss and that professional help is needed.

Most frequently, the person in need of help is taken to the emergency room of a general hospital or to the evaluation service of a general hospital or psychiatric institution where contact is made with a clinician who is able to perform a psychiatric assessment, who is familiar with the crisis unit and can arrange for the patient's admission.

THE NATURE OF REQUESTS FROM REFERRING CLINICIANS

The requests of referring clinicians are also multiple and include:

1. Evaluation of a patient and his family around a specific issue, e.g., an abortion
2. The stabilization of a patient's medication
3. Evaluation of a patient whose lack of intrapsychic controls or extrapsychic supports makes it impossible to perform a thorough evaluation on an outpatient basis
4. The arrangement of a disposition for a patient, e.g., a geriatric patient who has to be placed in a convalescent home
5. Detoxification of drug addict or alcoholic
6. Provision of definitive brief inpatient treatment for a broad spectrum of psychopathology
7. Tiding a patient through a stressful period, e.g., to maintain a chronic schizophrenic in a protective and supportive setting while a disturbed family situation is mediated.

Collaboration with referring sources is essential, and the ease with which complementary care can be arranged is an indication of how successfully a crisis unit has been integrated into the community and what value is attached to its services.

A crisis unit should serve as a convenient and available source of consultation, evaluation, and brief treatment, and complement longer-term outpatient treatment plans. For this to be achieved it is essential that the unit maintain good relations with other treatment facilities, private practitioners, and with the general public. This can be effected in the following ways:

The development of a good professional reputation through the provision of high-quality care; the education of both agencies and the public as to the services it offers; accessibility to patients in need of care (the unit should not have bureaucratic or academic restrictions that would hinder absorption of patients from the community, but rather should be seen by professionals and the public as being readily accessible); the provision of consultation and information to all professionals who contact the unit. This not only includes matters pertaining to admissions but can include advice towards resolving a variety of problems of a medical, psychiatric, or sociotherapeutic nature.

The Unit's Relationship to the Community

A close working relationship with appropriate members of the community is essential if the flow of patients from and back to the community is to be facilitated. It is helpful for staff members on a crisis unit to know people in numerous agencies in the community, and also for the agencies to be familiar with the design and workings of the crisis unit so that consultation can occur in both directions. Such reciprocity can be accomplished in a number of ways:

1. The staffing of the unit with people from various sociocultural backgrounds. One advantage of this is that it enables the unit to have as an immediate resource people who know the services available in different sections of the community. Secondly, it allows staff members who know a subculture to share information with the others on the unit; what is viewed as aberrant behavior by one subculture might be entirely within the norms of another. Finally, it affords residents of groups in the community the opportunity to acquire psychological skills which can be applied outside, e.g., in field stations and in community activities associations.

2. Visits by the staff to outside agencies. A staff member working with a patient may go with the patient, or alone, to investigate a possible follow-up disposition. This may involve a dinner at a halfway house or a commune, or a visit to the local welfare office. In turn, visits to the crisis unit by representatives of agencies allows the latter to see the unit and the services it provides, and promotes personal

contacts which may be helpful in arranging the disposition of patients.

3. Staff participation in training programs at outside agencies. This involves staff participation in training programs in areas such as drug dependence and alcoholism. This not only enables the staff to learn about reciprocal referral sources, such as a drug dependence facility or Alcoholics Anonymous, but provides a means whereby new ideas can be introduced into the functioning of the unit. People from these specialized agencies frequently appreciate an invitation to visit the unit to discuss the services they provide and to make recommendations about their preferences with regard to selection and referral of patients.

4. Visits by the staff to other hospitals. Clinicians can thus assess the strengths and shortcomings of facilities to which patients might be referred. The establishment of personal contacts between the crisis unit and other hospitals tends to promote better patient care when specific recommendations are made at the time of a patient's transfer.

5. The education of community groups by staff members. School, church and organized neighborhood community groups provide an excellent medium through which staff members can inform people about the services provided by the unit. The stigma associated with mental illness still exists in our society and contact with mental health professionals who demonstrate a problem-oriented approach can provide enlightenment and reassurance.

   The partial in-service training of community professionals such as clergy can contribute to the development of sophistication in the referral process. Clergymen who cannot recognize the severer forms of psychopathology may become overwhelmed by disturbed individuals who require psychiatric treatment. Conversely, they may underestimate their effectiveness with some people and refer them inappropriately for psychiatric treatment. The use of clergymen as consultants, often overlooked on more traditional psychiatric units, has been discussed by Hiltner (1972).

6. Attendance at unit meetings by the referring clinicians. This allows the staff to obtain first-hand information about a patient and enables the therapist to see what transpires with his patient during the hospitalization; this is frequently useful for the follow-up period. Good patient care is promoted when the therapists serving a community and the staff on a crisis unit get to know each other.

This undercuts the "we–them" syndrome which too often bedevils the therapist, the inpatient clinicians, and the patient.

7. Introduction of patients to therapists while on the unit. When a patient is referred to a therapist the first time, or when a change in therapists has occurred, it often helps for the therapist to have a brief initial meeting with the patient *on the unit*. This allows the patient the opportunity to form his own impressions about the therapist and the therapist an opportunity to assess how he may be of help.

8. Evaluation of referrals by nonpsychiatric groups. A referral for an evaluation is occasionally initiated by a nonpsychiatric source such as a law firm or a church group. The unit, because it emphasizes a limited stay and because it has access to a wealth of consultants, provides a unique service in that it can perform a comprehensive evaluation within days.

PROCESS OF CRISIS INTERVENTION

The Intake

An admission to the crisis unit generally begins with a phone call from a referring clinician. The call is taken by a staff member who gathers as much information as can be gleaned from a brief conversation, and then decides whether to accept the patient. Virtually all referrals are accepted for admission, except for assaultive, extremely regressed or heavily intoxicated patients. (See chapters on Detoxification and "Crises With Potential for Violence.") The staff member taking the referral always attempts to obtain at least the following:

1. Patient's name, address, and birth date
2. Name and address of next of kin
3. The nature of the presenting problem
4. The history of the presenting problem
5. Pertinent past history such as previous hospitalizations, psychoses, suicidal or homicidal behavior, and addictions to drugs or alcohol
6. Previous medical history
7. The name of the current therapist (if any)
8. The name of the referring clinician and his telephone number
9. How it is thought that the crisis unit can help.

The referring clinician is asked to summarize his impressions of the patient in a brief note and to have the patient or his relatives bring this to the unit. Should he indicate an interest in following the patient after discharge, he is told that the inpatient clinician will be in touch with him after the evaluation; he is also invited to attend rounds to share his ideas about the patient with the staff but is told that he should limit his personal contact with the patient to a few minutes at a time, and that he should not attempt to engage the patient in any discussion that may include decision making unless previously decided upon by the staff.

SPECIAL CONSIDERATIONS AROUND ADMISSION

1. The Suicide Attempt. When a patient has attempted suicide, we insist that he be cleared medically and that a note to that effect be attached to the referral note. Once the decision for admission is made, every endeavor is made to ensure that the patient comes directly to the unit—preferably accompanied by the clinician and a relative or friend—and that he is not allowed to go home and pack his belongings.

2. The Psychotically Disturbed Patient. The referring clinician is asked to ensure that the patient is medicated *before* he is brought to the unit. We generally recommend that Thorazine, 50mg IM, be given to assultive, agitated, restless or severly suicidal patients provided there are no medical contraindications, e.g. hypertension, old age. This often makes the work of the crisis staff easier and can also benefit the patient in making him more comfortable, and less likely to do anything that he might later regret; he will present himself in a way in which he is less likely to be labeled as "unmanageable." The unmanageable patient frequently engenders fear and distaste among the staff; often he will pick these feelings up and they may well serve to reinforce his behavior.

3. Serious Medical Problems. A thorough medical examination is a prerequisite for acceptance when patients with serious medical problems are admitted to the crisis unit through the emergency room.

4. Patients Under 18. Unless the patient is an emancipated minor, a parent or responsible family member or guardian over 18 must accompany him to sign him in.

5. Patients Who do not Speak or Understand English. It is very helpful if a relative or friend who knows English and is willing to act as a translator accompanies the patient to the unit.

6. Patients Who Have Children. Arrangements for the childrens' care (e.g., by an aunt) are made prior to admission.

   In general, if relatives are available they are encouraged to accompany the patient. Not only will they be needed for added information, but they may be of immediate help in calming the patient if he is excited or agitated. With elderly patients particularly, the presence of familiar faces often helps in dealing with a strange environment. However, relatives may overtly or surreptitiously provoke psychotic or acting-out behavior; in that case they are asked to leave after being told that they will be contacted after the patient has calmed down sufficiently to tolerate a visit.

THE PATIENT'S ARRIVAL ON THE UNIT

The general tone for the hospitalization is often set with the patient's first contact with a staff member. For this reason, a staff member approaches the patient as soon as he arrives on the unit, and after introducing himself and attending to the signing-in procedure, he proceeds to explain to the patient and his family the nature of the unit and how it functions.

Usually patients are told that it is hoped they will be discharged within a week. This is often a morale booster for the patient and his family and also helps them put their expectations into perspective. In addition, the patient is asked directly what he wants to accomplish during his stay. If his expectations seem reasonable, the staff member will confirm this to him and his family. The jobless, penniless alcoholic who claims that he only wishes to learn more about himself is told that this is an unreasonable proposition, and that unless he is willing to enlist the staff's aid in finding a job and seeking help for his drinking problem, he will not benefit from the hospitalization.

The significant family members are also asked what their expectations are. Often this task is not easy because of guilt, confusion, feelings of helplessness, or hidden expectations (e.g., to have an elderly parent placed in a convalescent home) which the family is entertaining. The staff approaches each admission in a straightforward, calm, and businesslike manner, at the same time conveying to the patient that an atmosphere of hope and warmth can be expected during the time he will spend on the unit.

GATHERING INFORMATION

The information necessary to evaluate and plan for treatment comes from many sources and is usually gathered by several staff members. Here, the interchangeability of their roles comes into play. The physical examination is, of course, performed by a physician, but the family history may be secured by a social worker, a psychiatrist, an aide, or a nurse.

The focus of information-gathering is on the circumstances that surround the admission and the social resources of the patient. The latter is most important in crisis work because of the urgency to begin formulating a discharge plan *when the patient is admitted.*

While questions about early family life and feelings towards family members are asked, these areas are not explored in the same depth *in every case*, as they would be on a long-term unit. Usually, a circumscribed history is what is needed. In a circumscribed history attention is paid mainly to the presenting problem and the patient's social matrix and mental status. (The mental status examination is described on page 52.) The only instance when a comprehensive psychiatric history is *routinely* obtained is with an adolescent or young adult.

The focus of detailed exploration should be information about living arrangements, contact with friends or relatives, and the patient's work situation. When a patient in crisis presents to a psychiatrist, the latter may be so impressed with the psychopathology that he may fail to note that the patient may have been living with auditory hallucinations for twenty years and is seeking help not because of his symptomatology but because the dwelling he has lived in for ten years is being torn down. The precipitant for the presentation is the threat of homelessness, and an evaluation of the patient's past preferences in terms of living arrangement and of his current needs in that regard will be what will contribute to an early and successful discharge from the unit.

The most useful sources of information generally include the patient and his family. In most cases the patient is the most reliable source of the nature of the crisis and of his past history. An interview with him will indicate where his strengths and weaknesses lie. It will also help in establishing a working alliance between him and a staff member. When the patient realizes that he is talking to a helpful and concerned person who encourages him to talk about painful aspects of his experience, he can begin developing a feeling of trust and confidence in the staff.

Formal interviews with the patient are generally valuable, but observing the way he relates to his family, friends, and other patients and staff members or the unit can provide a wealth of additional information about him. In particular, it reveals how he communicates his needs to others. An example of this would be a female patient who denies any feelings toward her husband but when informed that he has been asked to attend a joint interview the next day becomes anxious, cannot sleep, and spends an hour on her makeup and hair prior to his arrival.

The involvement of significant family members is invariably begun soon after the patient is admitted. Once it has been decided who to involve, the patient is usually encouraged to take the responsibility of contacting them. When, as occasionally occurs, he is reluctant to have a specific person come in, his resistance is dealt with directly, and if necessary, a staff member will contact the relative in question. The focus of information gathering from the family is on an evaluation of the patient and his crisis, and how the family can be involved in terms of discharge planning.

THE EVALUATION OF THE CRISIS

In general, there are few situations where the family cannot supply useful information. Corroborative and contradictory information are both significant. Parents, or a spouse, can be sources of pertinent facts, but occasionally siblings, grandparents, or distant relatives may be even more helpful. A distant relative who may have been intimately involved with the patient over a period of time is often in a better position to know a patient's strengths, weaknesses, and needs than anyone else.

Family involvement is mandatory for information gathering when the patient is too disorganized for a comprehensible history to be elicited, e.g., acute schizophrenic episodes, organic psychoses. It is essential in the case of an adolescent patient; here a developmental history can be provided by the family. Family involvement around an adolescent admission can serve another function, as the patient's behavior might be reflective of what is occurring in the parents' marriage. Frequently when an adolescent comes in for treatment, it is a signal that there is difficulty in the family of a serious nature.

FAMILY INVOLVEMENT IN DISCHARGE PLANNING

There are few situations where the family cannot be of help in discharge planning. Family members can rally around a depressed individual or provide companionship for a phobic patient so that he may negotiate otherwise impossible situations (e.g., trips to a supermarket, riding alone in elevators). Many situational disturbances cannot be resolved without continued involvement of family members after discharge. The family is absolutely essential in terms of discharge planning for some patients:

1. The Major Psychoses. Here family is often crucial in providing a suitable living arrangement, financial aid, and in making sure that the patient takes his medication.

2. Suicidal Patients. Where the risk of suicide will continue following discharge, meaningful family involvement is a prerequisite.
3. Organic Psychoses. When the family will continue to care for a patient with a chronic organic psychosis, their willingness to be involved in planning for discharge is mandatory. Decisions must be made as to who will be involved, when, and in what capacity. If, for example, an elderly lady with a senile psychosis insists on checking the plumbing in the basement every evening before retiring, all that may be necessary would be for someone to accompany her on her nightly mission.
4. Adolescent Patients. Adolescents can often not be relied on to follow up on various recommendations, e.g., to attend a birth control clinic, but if the parents are supportive and cooperative their resistances can be overcome.
5. Alcoholics. An assessment of the family is often overlooked in the treatment of alcoholics. Attention to the interpersonal dynamics will yield clues as to how a referral to Alcoholics Anonymous or other agencies might be accomplished.

A source of information that may complement the patient and his family is the outside therapist. When a patient is in psychotherapy at the time of the hospitalization, the therapist is always contacted. In the first place, he is usually a reliable source of historical information about the patient. Secondly, he can provide information about the current issues in the patient's life, including those related to the therapeutic relationship. When a patient who is in therapy attempts suicide, it frequently reflects to a greater or lesser degree what is transpiring in therapy. Finally, the therapist is the most reliable source of information about the medications that are being prescribed for the patient; in the case of an overdose he might know how much medication the patient had in his possession at the time.

The admitting clinician in most cases will provide a wealth of useful data when he calls to admit the patient. At times, however, it becomes necessary to contact him for clarification, as it often happens that the information provided at the time of the referral is insufficient or distorted. Anxiety, guilt, anger, or frustration might have been influencing his critical set. Or he may have been responding to external pressure, e.g., family, a supervisor, or the authorities, be they school, the law, or the church. In the days that follow the patient's admission the clinician has the opportunity to reappraise the situation more objectively and may be able to contribute effectively to the patient's management.

Other sources of information about the patient are workers, employers, and caseworkers. It is preferable to obtain the patient's consent to contact such people, but sometimes it may be in the patient's best interests to do so without consent. At times, many sources of information have to be tapped before it is possible to understand what is happening to a patient. Thus, someone who appears to be acutely schizophrenic may have been perfectly normal until he was surreptitiously given LSD the previous evening at a party. Similarly, a patient in a fugue state might have no recall of the events that led to admission. In this situation a sodium amytal interview will often provide the necessary information when it is not forthcoming from conventional sources. Thus, pragmatism must prevail in the acquisition of the information necessary for the proper assessment and treatment of the patients admitted to crisis units.

Once a patient has been accepted for admission to the unit, a staff member is immediately assigned the task of contacting the records room to ascertain whether records of previous contacts with the institution are available. If the patient has a chart, it is immediately sent to the unit to be reviewed. The information that can be extracted from a patient's old chart forms a template, which when added to the current evaluation, will provide an holistic assessment of him. From this a prognosis for the current illness and a speculative long-term prognosis can be made. The patient's strengths and weaknesses (and those of his family), his ways of coping with various situations, his response to hospitalizations and to medication can be more accurately formulated when his longitudinal life performance is evaluated in this way. The chart may contain adequate information about treatment at other institutions, and this will obviate the need for contacting those hospitals and waiting for records to arrive. Where there is a question of medical illness, arrangements are made to obtain records of the patient's medical history from other hospitals or private physicians.

In regions where crisis units are part of the state hospital system, the concept of *effective, episodic treatment* may one day become a reality once means are devised for rapid and accurate storage, transmission, and evaluation of information through computerization.

The Clinical Psychosocial Case History

Much that has been written about psychiatric interviewing has either tacitly or directly cautioned against the more task-oriented, question–answer type of interview (Sullivan, 1954; Stevenson, 1959). While it is agreed that where time allows, evaluation should take place over several sessions, the realities of time-limited crisis work preclude such an approach.

While a psychiatrist should review each history with the staff member who takes it, he seldom does the initial interview. Usually the patient's primary clinician does this since it will be his responsibility to integrate the therapeutic program and dictate the discharge summary.

The type of interview is determined by the age of the patient, the nature of the problem, and how much information has already been obtained from the patient's record or other sources. In all cases at least a circumscribed history is obtained.

An extensive psychiatric history, including a full developmental history, is obtained from adolescents and young adults; from some patients with major cognitive or affective disorders; and from patients when there is doubt about the diagnosis, e.g., the alcoholic who is suspected of drinking to cope with a longstanding schizophrenic disorder.

Even when information is available from records and other sources, having the patient relate the problem can serve as an organizing function for him as well as indicate to the clinician how clear the patient is about what he is trying to obtain through seeking help.

The functions of the psychosocial history on the crisis unit are multiple, and the relative importance of any one is determined by the time limitation and the tasks outlined by the unit. The interview outlined in Appendix A and discussed in this chapter can serve the following functions:

1. It provides information as to why the patient has come to the hospital and what he wants to get from the hospitalization. If a patient has been characterologically depressed for most of his life, why is it that he comes for treatment at age 40? Has there been a recent loss of some important support in the patient's life?

2. The information may provide important diagnostic information both psychiatrically and medically. Often psychiatric symptoms relate to an underlying medical problem. Also, despite the somewhat limited state of psychiatric nosology, certain diagnostic criteria have been defined (Robins *et al.*, 1972) which enable a psychiatrist to decide the appropriate role of psychotropic agents in the patient's treatment (See chapter on the use of psychotropic agents). A patient with recurrent mood swings presenting in an euphoric state with decreased sleep, grandiosity, flight of ideas, and pressured speech may, in the absence of a history of schizophrenia, benefit from the institution of lithium therapy, with further strain on the patient and his family avoided or minimized.

3. Information concerning the patient's social network is important in making realistic plans for preventing or minimizing further difficulties (Faris and Dunham, 1939; Leighton *et al.*, 1963). The effect of social disorganization in the genesis of suicidal behavior was described by Durkheim (1897) at the end of the last century. An individual's ability to survive in the community is greatly enhanced if the relative social supports are present. Often a patient may indeed have access to these, but as he becomes ill he withdraws, and people he has been close to in the past may be willing to aid at a time of crisis. However, the need has to be *communicated to them*, and there are intrapsychic factors which may interfere with a patient's ability to communicate his needs.

A typical example of this occurred when the relatives of a woman who was admitted because of a pathological grief reaction told us, "We seldom saw her after her husband died, but we felt she just wanted to be left alone for a while." This barrier is often a two-way one, and relatives of a patient may decide, for reasons that they are not always fully aware of, to avoid a situation which has personal meaning for them. The sister of another patient told us, "I had a miserable time after my father died and I've stayed away because

I thought I wouldn't be able to tolerate her crying all the time. Now that she's here I realize that I'm stronger than I thought I was and I want to help all I can."

4. The information can help in developing a realistic therapeutic plan. For instance, when it is discovered that a patient has to be hospitalized repeatedly because of his failure to take his medication, a regimen of intramuscular Prolixin Enanthate might be considered. In addition, certain prognostic factors have been defined in some psychiatric illnesses which if present may help relatives plan more realistically for the patient's future. For instance, Robins and Guze (1970) have shown that patients presenting with schizophrenia can be validly separated into poor prognosis and good prognosis groups. Features suggesting a good prognosis include the prominence of depressive symptoms, a family history of affective disorders, absence of a family history of schizophrenia, good premorbid adjustment, confusion, acute onset defined as less than six months of symptoms, precipitating factors, and concerns with dying and guilt. Poor prognosis is associated with an insidious onset (more than six months duration of symptoms), massive persecutory delusions, a hebephrenic clincial picture, clear sensorium, schizoid personality, family history of schizophrenia, and a striking emotional blunting.

5. The information gathered contributes to the interviewer's cognizance of the rich spectrum of normal and abnormal behavior. Clinicians are often amazed at how people with severely limited social and psychological resources can function often at a better level than those endowed with social assets. Judgment regarding this can be acquired only through careful and conscientious interviews with many patients. Payoffs often come at surprising times. For instance, one charming lady in her early seventies who was admitted with the diagnosis of "depression" seemed to be devoid of psychopathology until she was explicitly asked whether anyone was plotting against her, at which point she cordially stated, "Only my neighbors who are spraying my food with pigeon droppings, human blood and rat urine. Couldn't the doctor please help me get these cruel people arrested?"

6. The information gathered might be used for evaluative research of the effectiveness of treatment approaches used by the crisis unit with various types of patients. With the exception of the use of a few drugs (e.g., lithium carbonate in the treatment of manic–depressive illness) little can be said definitely about the efficacy of

the various treatment modalities offered by psychiatry. The information provided by the history can contribute to factor analytic studies of various therapies and of mental illnesses or symptom complexes. In addition, continuous assessment of the patient population being treated at a particular center is necessary if treatment programs relevant to the changing needs of a community are to be implemented. Where younger populations are being served, one can expect to see more acute schizophrenic breaks, drug psychoses secondary to hallucinogens, and problems pertaining to adolescence. If, on the other hand, the community being served comprises primarily the parents of a generation that has migrated to the suburbs, one may expect to see more geriatric problems, such as depressions secondary to retirement. In a slum area one can expect to see a greater incidence of alcoholism and drug addiction.

7. The interview allows the clinician and patient to get to know each other as human beings. Through this process hope can often be engendered in despairing situations. The interviewer acquires a feeling for how others with whom the individual has interacted have felt. He may detect a basic anger or a consuming neediness, leaving him feeling drained after the interview. The kindling of some quality of relatedness in an individual who at first seems entirely withdrawn, e.g., a severely depressed patient or a chronic schizophrenic, might be a key factor in helping him.

It cannot be emphasized enough that each crisis team must decide for itself what information it has the time to gather and how much information will be needed before decisions can be made. Ideally, most of the information in the comprehensive history discussed below should be obtained, but in a crisis situation this is often not feasible.

Computerized histories and mental status examinations like the ones included in the Appendix (Spitzer *et al.*, 1968, 1969, 1971) may aid information gathering and obtaining of records where facilities for processing them are available. By using such forms information gathered over several encounters could be made readily available, especially if there are mutual arrangements between various centers and states.

The history-taking to be presented in the remainder of this chapter (see Appendix A) represents an outline for a comprehensive history of a crisis unit. It provides, in addition, the substrate from which a circumscribed history can be condensed.

The comprehensive history is generally accomplished in one and one half to two hours. While it is presented in a chronological manner, in practice information relevant to any one area is often obtained while discussing another. For the sake of convenience, is is divided into four parts:

1. Description of the Patient. The demographic information needed on every patient includes age, sex, marital status, occupation, religion, race, children, and living arrangement. Demographic information is important in both psychiatric practice and research. Should the patient be hospitalized again, any changes may be a sign of stresses he has experienced or gains he has made since his last hospitalization.

   Discrepancies between chronological age and physical appearance might suggest that life has taken an undue toll of the patient.

   Ethnographic data can be used to assess the support a patient may have in the community. The extended Italian family is but one example of a social access often helpful in the treatment of a depressed patient.

   Finally, the demographic data is and has been helpful in the statistical study of behavior such as suicide, e.g., the knowledge that suicidal risk is greater among the divorced and widowed was arrived at both by the analysis of demographic data and by clinical experience.

2. Chief Complaint. The patient's own words are used to describe what he sees as the problem bringing him to the crisis unit. If relatives or friends see his problem differently, a notation to that effect is made.

3. History of the Present Illness. No matter when the history relevant to the present illness is obtained in the interview, it should be presented chronologically in as concise a manner as possible. Information relating to the onset of the symptoms, and how they have influenced the various spheres of the patient's life—social, academic, occupational, sexual, physiological, and familial—should be obtained.

   Patients are often unable or unwilling to describe clearly the course of their symptoms or to reveal what is really bothering them. Direct questions about changes in interpersonal relationships, about sex, and about money are often necessary before insight can be gained about the patient's problem. With a married patient, for instance, it is always important to inquire about infidelity. Adolescents should be tactfully questioned about menstruation, masturbation, and the nature of their sexual orientation.

   Feelings common to many crisis patients are those of shame or guilt, and a degree of alleviation of such pressures can be enormously beneficial. Myths and taboos about sexual practices still abound in society; it is amazing, for instance, how many children are still raised to believe that masturbation causes sterility or insanity. When guilt which is based on irrational or simply uninformed beliefs is disclosed, straightforward reassurance can be therapeutic. Some adolescents who have abortions are deeply concerned about their ability to conceive again, and simple reassurance will be beneficial once the fantasies about the procedure have been explored.

Obstacles are often encountered in the interview when trying to get an accurate assessment of the patient's resources. By and large, patients are quite willing to discuss the intimate details of their sex lives, but abhor discussing their finances. Some of the reasons are obvious and relate to the patient's life situation, his needs and those of his family. Patients will often consciously give false information. A grandmother who has sizable blue chip holdings on the stock market but leans heavily on her family for emotional support might hide the details of her fortune as a way of controling her children's and grandchildren's behavior toward her. We have seen such an individual create a tremendous fuss and claim penury when the issue of paying to see a private therapist was raised.

Many times, however, the resistance to discussing income or savings is deeply rooted in the patient's unconscious. It is common knowledge that economic factors play an enormous role in peoples' lives, yet judging from the anecdotal nature (Bergler, 1970) and paucity of the literature of this topic, it is clear that very little is understood about the psychology of money and how it relates to psychodynamics and psychopathology. In any event, it is important to try to get an idea about the patient's finances and his attitudes about money. It is also incumbent on the crisis worker to know something about the economic structure of the patient's subculture, e.g., welfare, unemployment, disability compensation, so that the economic forces working for and against the patient can be included in the assessment of his functioning.

Included in the history of the present illness should be explicit data relating to appetite, weight change, and alteration of sleep patterns. It is important to ask about difficulty in falling asleep, awakening during the night or restless sleep, early morning awakening, hypersomnia, and whether there has been a change in the nature, content, or frequency of dreams (it is often overlooked that severely depressed patients tend to stop dreaming).

Suicidal and homicidal thoughts or impulses must be thoroughly assessed. Changes in the patient's interest in and attitude towards his family, friends, work, or school should be noted, and patterns of drug and alcohol use should be carefully documented. The latter is usually a difficult task and often requires detailed questioning. The quantity and type of intoxicants being ingested has to be carefully assessed as well as the setting in which the ingestion occurs, e.g., does an alcoholic drink alone, does an adolescent smoke marijuana only when pressured to do so by friends. It is equally important to determine what effect the intoxicant has on the patient, both from a psychological and a medical standpoint, e.g., has a patient with a history of alcohol consumption ever experienced an alcoholic psychosis or has he ever been jaundiced. Users of intoxicants are frequently extremely skilled in hiding the presence or extent of an addiction so it is mandatory to inquire specifically about each drug among those commonly abused. A frequent pitfall is overlooking a barbiturate, amphetamine, or analgesic (e.g., Darvon) habituation.

The response of the patient's associates to the changes that occurred as he became ill are also important (e.g., was he fired from work). Information gathered in the mental status examination may be included in the history of the present illness when developing a longitudinal picture. If, for example, the patient acknowledges hallucinations, derealization, depersonalization, ideas of reference, or paranoid ideation, the time of onset should be included here. Putting the patient's present psychiatric problems in the context of his previous psychiatric treatment is best placed in this part of the history. The previous psychiatric history should include details about all known previous consultations, hospitalizations, or outpatient therapies as well as somatic therapy (psychotropic medication, EST) and the patient's response to it.

4. Personal History. In almost a biographical manner the development of the patient from birth and infancy to the present state is traced. Depending on the circumstances of treatment and what information has been obtained before, modification of the history can occur. There is probably no better way to develop an understanding of individual psychodynamics as well as developing a supportive relationship with the patient than by carefully and interestedly listening to a patient recount his life story. For many, this experience will be new and will not only function in an organizing manner but will also set the patient's problem in a perspective

which may enable him to develop some insight into maladaptive patterns, as well as alert the interviewer to his primary defensive patterns. The patient's strengths will also come through. Although many patients may present with the acute symptoms of depression, social functioning is varyingly affected, suggesting that there are other factors affecting his social role performance. Often, the areas found to be most profoundly affected are those involving an individual's closest interpersonal relationships (Weissman *et al.*, 1971). There might be significantly less impairment at work than at home. Friction in interpersonal relationships seems to increase as a function of the closeness of these relationships. It is the interviewer's task to define the individual's strength as well as his weaknesses.

It has often been said that if anything a man learns from history, it is that he doesn't learn from history. A careful look at what a patient has done and can do is often much more important than what he says he can do and will do and never has. Although this part of the history sometimes seems an immense task, most of our staff (with the proper supervision) find that they could do it in forty-five minutes to an hour.

Birth and Early Childhood. Often, a lot can be obtained from a patient about his own birth and infancy. The achievement of the milestones (walking, talking, etc.), which may serve to indicate his intellectual endowment, will usually have been mentioned in the family. Difficulty before, during, or after a delivery can foreshadow not only later psychiatric difficulty but neurological disease as well. German measles during the first three months of pregnancy resulting in mental retardation, or trauma due to the use of forceps resulting in minimal brain damage are but two of numerous psychiatric problems seen on a crisis unit that relate to birth.

The patient's birth order and ordinal relationship to the birth of his siblings is important in assessing how much attention was allotted the individual during this critical time of early childhood. Maternal depression during or after the pregnancy may suggest the mother's response to the birth. Childhood symptoms which may have remnants in adult life are important: head banging, bed wetting phobias, stuttering, and speech disorders should be asked about.

Family Life. An investigation of the patient's relation to family members while growing up is important for all patients, but especially adolescents. To be loved and appreciated in one's home is a gift which is often invaluable in preparing a person for rejections or losses in later life. A history of early parental loss through death or divorce is not infrequently found in the history of patients who later become susceptible to depression (Brown, 1961; Beck, 1967). A lack of security in the family situation might leave the person feeling vaguely insecure throughout his life, and prone to the loss of self-esteem. Indeed, as Wordsworth states, "The child is father of the man." The patient should be specifically asked to describe his father and mother, tell whether either favored any of their children over others, and who he feels he resembles. Often the patient will describe his parents briefly as "my father was warm but very authoritarian, and my mother was busy all the time with her housework." Family constellations, e.g., the father being distant and detached and the mother being closely binding and intimate in families of male homosexuals (Bieber, 1965), have been described. Particularly important in crisis work is clearly defining what role relatives play in the patient's present life. They are often valuable supports and can be helpful in deciding on the best disposition.

Academic Development.   A record of the person's progress at school can serve as a sensitive barometer to other things going on in his life. An adolescent's academic failure after several years of above average performance may indicate intrapsychic conflict or family turmoil. Specific questions about what is going on at home are then indicated. Are his parents arguing or talking of separating? A schizophrenic who presents at age twenty-one with a history of being a valedictorian of his high school class but who has over the subsequent three years shown a decline in his academic performance has a worse prognosis than the one who was an honors student right up until the time that he became ill. An intelligent black adolescent in a ghetto situation may present with a history of antisocial behavior following frustration in the classroom or at home if little value was placed on the talent that he perceived himself to have.

Interpersonal Relationships.   Defining a person's social network is not as easy as it may seem at first. A person may glibly answer that indeed he has "many" friends, but when questioned more carefully, he may not be able to mention one by name. One must ask when and how often he sees his friends. Does he belong to any organizations at school or in his community? The structures of such relationships vary significantly among the social classes. A lower-class Italian laborer's closest relationships may be with his extended family, whereas a lower-class black patient's closest relationships may be with his neighbors. An upper-class white patient's school album may remain his closest support. It is often not as important who the patient has as support but how close, reliable, and accessible they are in times of difficulty. Communicating to these individuals the patient's needs may be the primary defined task in a crisis situation.

A change in the character of interpersonal relationships is often a sign of psychiatric difficulty. A seventeen-year-old girl presenting with gradual withdrawal from friends and preoccupation with her own fantasies often indicates an impending schizophrenic episode. It is worthwhile to conceptualize a patient's personality as a mosaic of strengths and weaknesses. Although a patient may be moderately depressed throughout his life, his ability to make and sustain friendships may protect him from an emotional breakdown.

Religious Development. A brief (one- or two-sentence) description of the role of religion in the patient's life is helpful. Religious rituals or delusions may be a manifestation of a neurosis or psychosis, but religion may also serve an integrative function. Durkheim (1897) pointed out the role of religion in the prevention of suicide. If a patient is or has been interested in religious activities, this may benefit him in the future.

Psychosexual Development. Sexual development, activity, and fantasy must be asked about not only because this information will help in the assessment of the case, but also because it conveys to the patient the sense that openness is encouraged. As mentioned, the alleviation of guilt or fear in this area, e.g., mastubatory guilt, may often be of enormous therapeutic value. Questions about abortion, menstruation, the ability to achieve orgasm and the attitude towards pregnancy must be specifically asked about with an emphasis on uncovering the emotional correlates. Sexual functioning is a sensitive and reliable guideline to an individual's emotional well being and is an essential part of the history.

Occupational History. Ability to function at work, like ability to function in interpersonal relationships or at school, is another accurate reflection of emotional well-being. If a forty-five-year-old patient has been able to hold a job for twenty years, his ability to return to work from the hospital and support himself is obviously greater than one of comparable age who has held thirty jobs in the same period. Sometimes the lack of consistent work outside the home may be the cause of a depression in a woman who feels that her ability is being wasted. Again, it is important to get an assessment of the patient's income and to get a rough assessment of his expenses, remembering that patients frequently distort information about this in both directions. Financial concerns or difficulties frequently play a part in the development of acute psychiatric symptomatology.

Living Arrangement.   Not infrequently a patient will present because of some difficulty in his living arrangement. An elderly person who relocates may become depressed and even develop symptoms of senility. The loss of familiar faces, stores, and churches may precipitate a feeling of disorientation. Object constancy is very important in the lives of schizophrenics, and a recent, impending or imagined change in his living arrangement can precipitate a decompensation which might heal rapidly once constancy is restored.

A young married couple who have moved five times in the first year of their marriage suggests the possibility that all is not well with their marriage, even though the ostensible complaint is about the plumbing or the neighbors. People often move with the fantasy that they will leave all their difficulties behind them. Relocations are always significant from the standpoint of why they were effected and what the effects are. There may be obvious reasons why people move, but often there are other reasons of which the patient is only dimly aware: the revelation of these may be of help to him.

Where a patient lives is something he holds very much in common with those who live with him, and it is not uncommon for a domino effect to occur where the gas gets turned off for non-payment, mother lets fly at father, who in turn criticizes daughter, whose recourse then becomes a suicide gesture as a form of protest. Warmth, food, and other taken-for-granted provisions in a home enormously affect emotional well being.

Family History.   Questions concerning the ages of family members, their occupations and states of health (and circumstances and time of death, if dead) are important. Where the relatives live and how frequently they are seen are clues to their supportive role. Schizophrenic disorders and affective disorders seem to follow familial patterns, although the roles of genetics and environment are yet to be defined. A history of these disorders as well as alcoholism, neurological disease, and epilepsy must be obtained. Asking about the occurrence of divorce in a family might help in determining a picture of the interpersonal stability in the family; a lack of the latter suggests a high prevalence of psychopathology.

Medical History. Less medical history is obtained from a psychiatric patient than from a medical one, but all operations, trauma, and illness should be noted as well as the emotional responses to them. A history of real or symbolic losses of procreative power, e.g., the response to a prostate operation, is important. It is also essential to inquire about medications being used, e.g., some antihypertensive agents are capable of causing severe depression.

History of Drug Use. A significant challenge to the clinician is to obtain a reasonably accurate history of alcohol and drug use from psychiatric patients. Since most patients who do indulge do not reveal the extent of their use of intoxicants, it is important to keep intoxicant use in mind, carefully observe the patient's appearance, and ask questions of relatives in order to get an accurate assessment. Although drug use is prevalent among adolescents, there are many middle-aged people who "turn on." Drugs such as Darvon, Sominex, and Librium are frequently abused by middle-aged persons. If a positive history of drug use is obtained, the patient should be asked for a list of the different types and relative frequencies of drugs he has used. If a positive history is obtained for alcohol, then drug use, particularly barbiturates, should be inquired about.

Military History. This should never be overlooked as persons with psychiatric illness may first experience difficulty in the service, and the nature of the disturbance often suggests much about a person's ability to react to stress, his response to authority figures, to the atmosphere of violence, and to some of the homosexual undercurrents that prevail in military life. It is, therefore, important to inquire about classification (if rejected, why), circumstances of discharge, adjustment to regimented military life, participation in active combat, and the emotions aroused by combat.

Legal History. These questions should deal with the patient's experiences, past and present, with the law. Has he ever been brought to trial or imprisoned? If so, why? On a crisis unit it is important to know whether a patient is pending trial. If so, it must be determined what relationship the legal problem has to the psychiatric presentation.

Psychiatric History. Previous psychiatric hospitalization and outpatient consultations, and treatments must be inquired about. A regressed schizophrenic with a history of twelve previous hospitalizations, all of which lasted in excess of 6 months is unlikely to benefit from a brief hospitalization.

THE MENTAL STATUS EXAMINATION

A task that many nonmedical psychiatric professionals are reluctant to undertake is the mental status examination. It is felt by some that it is a specialized examination, similar to a neurological examination, which can be effectively performed only by a physician. Others feel that it is an invasion of the psychiatrist's domain to perform it, and for this reason shy away. It is also thought of as an examination in the academic sense, that a patient either passes or fails.

A major preoccupation is that once a patient is persuaded to reveal his disordered thinking or violent impulses, he will lose control and immediately act on the thoughts and feelings. Many clinicians are hesitant to ask a patient specifically about suicidal ideas for fear that if they do not already exist, the examiner will instill these thoughts in the patient's mind. In this regard, it has been demonstrated that inquiring about suicidal ideation does not precipitate suicidal behavior. Some clinicians believe that asking a patient about hallucinations or delusions might embarrass him; this is seldom the case as most patients feel relieved when able to share their disturbing innermost thoughts with others.

Initially, everyone experiences some anxiety about doing a mental status examination. It takes time and experience to master the skills necessary to structure the examination, to feel comfortable asking questions about highly charged topics such as suicide and homicide, and to develop a technique whereby much of the information that has to be included in the examination can be obtained from sources other than the formal mental status examination.

During the psychiatric interview, disorders of mood such as manic elation or retarded depression, disorders of thinking such as looseness of associations or neologisms, disorders of perception such as hallucinations or illusions, and disorders of behavior such as restlessness or catatonia might become manifested. Observation of the patient on the unit and information gathered from family or friends will usually contribute further to an understanding of the patient's mental apparatus.

When the mental status examination is performed one is therefore armed with a considerable background of information that will help one to organize in his mind which areas must be focused on and which need to be only cursorily explored or possibly omitted. It is, however, essential when documenting the findings to include all the relevant facts regardless of where they are obtained.

In terms of organizing the examination into a concise package it is therefore necessary to have a structured model, such as that which is described in Appendix B. But the sequence of questions and the emphasis or deemphasis on certain areas must be tailored to the patient. The following is a brief discussion of the mental status examination presented in Appendix B.

1. General Appearance. The first assessment is of the patient's level of consciousness. In this regard it is important to determine whether the patient is alert and communicative or unresponsive. Lack of response can be due to the withdrawal that is characteristic of catatonia, but is often the result of neurological conditions such as toxic states (e.g., drug overdose, acute alcoholic intoxication), encephalitis, and cerebral trauma.

   A description of the patient's appearance and dress is important as it will indicate not only something about how he cares for himself or is looked after, but it may also give a clue to his concept of himself.

   Anxiety may be manifested in many ways, such as fidgeting, constant recrossing of legs, moving about in the chair, difficulty in articulating clearly due to a dry mouth, or having to interrupt the interview to go to the toilet.

   Any peculiar mannerisms, twitches, compulsive acts, or unusual posturing should be noted by the interviewer. An ataxic or "drunken" gait may indicate alcohol or drug intoxication, or may be the manifestation of a disease affecting the nervous system.

2. Activity Level. The patient's activity level serves as an important indicator of his mood. The person with an *agitated depression* will typically pace the floor and wring his hands while accusing himself of sins so horrible that no punishment is too cruel. The patient with a *retarded depression* may sit quietly while gazing despairingly at the floor. A *manic* will often move rapidly around the room recounting fantastic adventures, and may provoke laughter from the interviewer.

3. Orientation. To determine how well a patient is oriented, it is necessary to ask him his name, the time, the day, the month, and the year, and where he is. Except for very confused psychiatric patients, these questions can usually be answered with accuracy. Patients with organic brain syndromes, such as those due to senility or intoxication from drugs or alcohol, may have much more diffi-

culty. Usually the sense of time is the first to go, then place, and finally person.

The mechanism underlying disorientation is *memory distur-bance.* However, disorientation is traditionally distinguished from memory disturbance and for the sake of consistency this is adhered to here.

4. Memory Disturbance. In psychiatric illness, difficulty with recent memory is more significant than difficulty with past memory. A senile patient may have a poor memory for recent events but might be able to remember his childhood in detail. The loss of recent memory is strongly suggestive of an organic brain syndrome. A good way to test it is to give the patient the names of three objects to remember at the beginning of the mental status examination (e.g., wall, key, pen) and to ask at the end of the interview whether he can remember them.

5. General Intelligence. Assessment of a patient's intelligence is at best crude, and his performance may be influenced by cultural factors. However, asking a patient simple questions, such as how many days there are in a week or to name the four seasons of the year, does give an indication; also performance of simple mathematics (e.g., what is four plus four).

   Some clinicians find it helpful to administer the information sub-test of the Weschler Adult Intelligence Scale. This test has a high correlation with a full-scale I.Q. but, nonetheless, should be deemed just a screening test. Clinical experience has shown that a high score on this test indicates high intelligence more reliably than a low score indicates low intelligence. Psychiatric and cultural factors may affect a patient's response to any test aimed at determining intelligence. A knowledge of what a patient has been able to accomplish, given his subculture, may give one more reliable lead than what can be derived from a formal test.

   Two parameters of intelligence that can always be rapidly assessed are the quality of an individual's vocabulary and his fund of information. This determination can occur during the psychiatric interview as well as during more informal contacts that one might have with a patient.

6. Mood and Affect. Mood represents a sustained emotion while affect represents a brief, transient response. The motor concomitants of mood are described under Activity Level, but the patient should be explicit asked if he feels elated or depressed. A smiling counte-nance does not mean that a patient is not depressed and, in fact,

can be a dangerous sign in a depressed person as it may serve to hide his difficulties.

Appropriateness of affect is an important determinant of psychopathology. Schizophrenics may laugh or smile while recounting sad aspects of their lives. Patients who have a chronic history of mental illness (particularly schizophrenia) or a long history of institutionalization may present with almost no emotional response; this is called "flat affect." Quickly fluctuating emotion, especially where there is no obvious provocation, suggests an organic brain syndrome.

7. Ambivalence. Everyone is ambivalent to some extent about interpersonal relationships. A young wife might get angry at her husband because he smokes, but she still loves him because he is basically kind and is a good companion and provider. A schizophrenic, however, may feel hate and love at the same time and seem confused about how to respond.

8. Delusions. A delusion is a false belief which a patient clings to despite objective evidence and logic to the contrary. Delusions may take several forms, but the three most commonly seen are persecutory, grandiose, and depressive delusions.

Patients with *persecutory delusions* may feel that people or organizations such as the C.I.A., the F.B.I., or just a vague "they" are after them. Such patients often have *ideas of reference,* e.g., while walking down a street they may believe that everyone is watching them or talking about them. In paranoid schizophrenia, persecutory delusions are often combined with *delusions of influence,* in which, for instance, a patient may feel that electric beams from another planet are controlling his behavior.

Grandiose delusions are encountered in manics, schizophrenics, and in some organic states. A manic may feel that he is the wealthiest man in the world and, in fact, may be brought for care because his wild spending attracted the attention of his family.

Severely depressed patients often present with *depressive delusions* involving guilt, sin, impoverishment, hopelessness, worthlessness, or illness. They may feel that they are the worst of all possible people and should be punished for their sins and for the evil they have brought on their families and on the world.

9. Hallucinations. An hallucination is a false sensory perception which arises in the absence of any external stimulus. Hallucinations take on a variety of forms. The most frequent are auditory (hearing) and visual (sight) hallucinations. Olfactory (smell), gustatory (taste), tac-

tile (touch), and kinesthetic (position sense) hallucinations also occur but are relatively rare.

Once the presence of hallucinations has been verified, it is important to evaluate what sensory modalities are involved, what the intensity of the hallucinations is, how the patient reacts to them, and whether he believes them to be real or has some understanding as to their origin. For instance, a depressed schizophrenic who admits to hearing his mother's voice calling to him from the grave may be a serious suicide risk. Hallucinations occur in a variety of illnesses, including schizophrenia, organic psychoses, and toxic psychoses such as those caused by LSD or alcohol.

10. Concept Formation. The ability to abstract should be tested in every patient. Lack of this ability, which is referred to as concrete thinking, has been described by Goldstein (1959) as being an important characteristic of brain-damaged individuals. A normal individual is said to possess the ability to think on two different levels: the concrete and the abstract. When one's thoughts reflect a response to the immediate experience of things and situations, he is said to think concretely. The ability to transcend from the immediate sensory impression to a symbolic interpretation is called the ability to abstract. People with brain damage secondary to many causes often lose this capacity. However, chronic schizophrenics may also demonstrate this defect. To test for it, one generally asks for the interpretation of a familiar proverb, e.g., a "a rolling stone gathers no moss." In addition to assessing the ability to abstract, this gives a patient with a thought disorder another opportunity to reveal his haphazard thinking. One acutely schizophrenic patient responded to the proverb about glass houses by saying that "the glass is obviously the secret and that meaning relates also to God and sex. . . ."

11. Phobias. Patients should be questioned about the presence of phobias or irrational fears. These often have special names such as hydrophobia (fear of water), claustrophobia (fear of enclosed spaces), agoraphobia (fear of open spaces), acrophobia (fear of heights), or thanatophobia (fear of death). Knowing the names (which are usually derived from Greek) is not as important as identifying the phobia if present and ascertaining to what extent it interferes with a person's functioning.

12. Hypochondriacal Ideation. Concerns about bodily function are found in many people from normal to psychotic but some patients, particularly the depressed or hysterical, will go from physician to physician seeking help for headaches, stomachaches, etc., which

have no organic basis. Hypochondriacal complaints should not be confused with *psychophysiological disorders* or with *somatic delusions*. *Psychophysiological disorders* are organic dysfunctions, such as ulcerative colitis, where emotional factors presumably underlie the organic illness. *Somatic delusions* are typically discovered in the psychotically depressed patient, who may believe that his brain has turned into sawdust or that his body is full of worms.

The following is a glossary of the terms that most frequently cause difficulty to clinicians who are unfamiliar with the mental status examination:

Ambivalence: The simultaneous existence of contradictory emotions towards the same person or experience.

Anhedonia: The inability to experience pleasure.

Apathy: Remarkable reduction or absence of emotion in situations usually provocative of feelings.

Blocking: Abrupt cessation of a train of thought.

Catatonic Stupor: Total unresponsiveness based not on organic factors or a profound depression, but rather a complete withdrawal of a patient from his environment.

Circumstantiality: Central thought is lost in a plethora of details.

Clang Associations: The association of certain words because of sound similarity, e.g., sang, bang, rang.

Compulsions: Repeated acts over which the patient feels he has no control, e.g., turning the gas on and off to make sure it's off.

Condensation: Fusion of more than two ideas or concepts.

Concreteness: Taking everything said literally.

Delusions: False beliefs which exist despite evidence to the contrary.

Depersonalization: A reported feeling of being apart from oneself and looking at oneself like an actor on a stage. A loss of the sense of one's personal identity.

Derealization: The sensation that the world around one is losing its real qualities.

Déjà Vu: The feeling that what is being experienced occurred before in one's life, e.g., walking through a building in a city one has never been in before and finding it familiar.

Echolalia: Meaningless repetition of another's words.

Echopraxia: Meaningless repetition of another's movements.

Euphoria: An extreme feeling of well being.

Flat Affect: Very little or no modulation of emotional response.

Flight of Ideas: Thoughts rapidly passing through a patient's mind.

Hallucinations: Sensations experienced without the appropriate external stimulus in the waking state, e.g., hearing voices when no one is present.

Illusions: A misinterpretation of a real external situation, e.g., the shadow of a tree may be seen as a person.

Inappropriate Affect: Emotional response that is not consistent with what is being discussed, e.g., laughing when talking of one's father's death.

Lability of Affect: Rapidly shifting or unstable affect.

Loose Associations: Lack of logical connection between contiguous elements of speech and thinking.

Obsession: Recurring irrational thoughts intruding into the patient's mind without his control—often associated with compulsive behavior in an attempt to ward off the thoughts and anxiety accompanying them.

Perseveration: Repetition of a particular action or verbalization without apparent external stimulus.

Phobia: Irrational, excessive fear of a particular object or situation.

Psychomotor Retardation: A slowing down of both psychological and physical activity.

Tangential Speech: Digressing from a thought begun without returning to it.

Verbigeration: Constant repetition of meaningless words or phrases.

THE MEDICAL EVALUATION

While most patients presenting on the crisis unit have totally unremarkable medical evaluations, there are others whose symptomatology is either 1) a manifestation of an underlying organic process or 2) a reaction to a preexisting medical illness. Examples of the first include derealization and depersonalization occurring in temporal lobe epilepsy, loose associations and confusion occurring with encephalitis, and depression occurring with lead toxicity. An example of reaction to a medical symptom is a depressive presentation in a woman who has a breast lump which she suspects is malignant, has not told anyone, including her family and doctor, and has as a result become anxious and depressed.

The first step in a thorough medical evaluation is to obtain a medical and surgical history. Thereafter a complete physical examination should be performed. It is best to do this shortly after the patient is admitted so that psychotropic medication can be started immediately if necessary. Except as an emergency, for medicolegal reasons, one cannot give a patient medication on an inpatient unit before he has had a physical examination.

There are several ways of delegating the task of the physical examination on a crisis unit. If psychiatrists are available on a full-time basis (as opposed to just consultative), it should be their responsibility. If, however, there are no full-time psychiatrists, then the unit has to insist that whoever is referring the patient either personally perform the physical examination or arrange for it to be done by a colleague. The best solution is for a crisis unit to have a part-time internist as medical back-up. He is then responsible for physical examinations on all patients admitted during the day, as well as being a consultant on medical problems. For after-hour medical coverage, a crisis unit should have either a psychiatrist from the institution or a part-time internist on hand to examine the patient shortly after admission. Where access to a physician for medical back-up is difficult or impossible, the physical examination could be performed by a physician's associate or a nurse clinical practitioner.

All patients admitted should have routine complete blood counts, VDRL's, blood glucose estimations, and urinalyses. In addition, facilities should be on hand for serum lithium estimations, roentgenography, and electroencephalography. An EKG machine should be available for use by the crisis unit, particularly for patients over the age of forty-five who are being evaluated for antidepressant or phenothiazine treatment. If phenothiazines or antidepressants are to be prescribed, liver function tests should be performed prior to commencement of the medication.

Other elective tests frequently performed are a pregnancy test, thyroid studies, and specialized neurological examinations such as skull x rays, EEG's and brain scans. Hypochondriacal patients, or patients with somatic delusions, can run a crisis team ragged. Questions pertaining to special tests, examinations, or procedures should be carefully evaluated by the psychiatrist who will then decide whether a referral or consultation is indicated.

Evaluation of Suicidal and Homicidal Potential

The assessment of a patient's suicidal or homicidal potential is an important part of an evaluation but for many mental health professionals, including psychiatrists, it engenders anxiety. This may be because decisions made following these evaluations include perhaps the ultimate in responsibility—other peoples' lives.

It is often difficult for the staff to accept the impossibility of making absolute statements about patient's suicidal or homicidal potential. No more than an educated guess can be made based on what epidemiological evidence there is available. We do not and cannot have complete control over people, and there will be patients who remain suicidal to one degree or another throughout their lives. As Eugene Bleuler states in his classical 1911 monograph *Dementia Praecox and the Group of Schizophrenias,* given a population of schizophrenics, a few *will commit suicide,* but to keep those with that recurrent potential throughout their lives institutionalized is unkind (Bleuler, 1950). Suicidal patients are frequently admitted to the crisis unit, and many are discharged with some uncertainty about their imminent or longterm potential for suicide. It is a mark of a mature clinician that he can function with this uncertainty, and that he knows which patients are potentially suicidal and what circumstances aggravate the risk.

One of the functions of a crisis unit is to help patients who would traditionally be deemed candidates for long-term hospitalization stay out of long-term hospitals. Even though the number of hospitalizations may be increased in this manner, the actual number of hospital days is greatly reduced. The patient is often saved from the toll that long-term institutionalization takes particularly in the form of regression, and financial cost. A crisis unit, because of its structure and its goals, can function effectively and inexpensively as a base for the *episodic treatment* of intermittently or chronically suicidal patients.

One of the goals of a crisis unit is to enable such patients to function in the community using supports available there to sustain them. Durkheim (1897) in relating suicide rates to the level of social integration, contended that in great crisis the rates of suicide fall because society is more strongly integrated and individuals participate more actively in the social life of the community. The lower suicide rates among Catholics and Jews is attributed to the fact that religion closely integrates people into the collective life. This information is helpful when working with suicidal patients who live in communities that are disintegrating, be they disorganized ghettos with a high degree of anomie or elderly people who have moved from an "urban village" to a skyscraper apartment, where they feel lost in a sea of identical-looking apartment rooms.

The task of the crisis unit is in many cases to define what group support, be it dyadic or greater, the depressed suicidal individual can get so that he does not feel so lost, alone, and without support and security.

Studies of suicidal and homicidal behavior have identified some epidemiological correlates of self-destructive behavior and are helpful in assessing a person's suicide potential.

EVALUATION OF SUICIDE RISK

1. Marital Status. Divorced or separated people comprise a disproportionate percentage of suicides (Farberow *et al.*, 1965), and widowed individuals show especially high rates (Sainsburg, 1955). Their self-inflicted deaths cluster in the first years of bereavement (MacMahon *et al.*, 1965).

   The lowest rates appear to be among the married, especially those with children. The rates for single people average twice those of the married, and the rates for the divorced or widowed are from four to five times higher than the married (Hendin, 1967).

2. Presence of Physical Illness. There is a high correlation between physical illness and suicidal behavior (Dorpat *et al.*, 1968). The presence of a disabling or painful illness, such as cancer, particu-

larly in someone who was robust, presents a considerable risk.

3. Depression. All patients whose mood is depressed should be carefully questioned as to their suicide potential (Susser, 1968).

4. Severe Insomnia. Regular early morning wakening with restlessness indicates a high risk.

5. Correlation to Gender. The risk of suicide is higher among men (Susser, 1968), although women may gesture more. Men will frequently make more lethal attempts using violent means, whereas women seem to prefer to overdose. The percentage of males and females are 70 and 30 respectively for successful suicides, while the percentage for attempted suicides are nearly the reverse, 31 and 69 respectively (Farberow and Shneidman, 1965).

6. Schizophrenia. Clinical experience suggests that suicidal behavior is much more difficult to predict in schizophrenics (Farberow and Shneidman, 1957). A combination of a depressed mood, a thought disorder, and suicidal ideation is ominous. Especially ominous are "command" hallucinations telling the patient to kill himself, or the hallucination of the voice of a departed loved one beckoning the patient to join him in the world beyond.

7. Alcoholism and Drug Addiction. Clinical experience shows that suicidal behavior is difficult to predict in alcoholics (Farberow and Shneidman, 1957) and in drug addicts. While an addict or alcoholic may not consciously elect to kill himself, his judgment may become impaired to the point where he might, for instance, take an excess of barbiturates in order to sleep. In susceptible individuals alcohol or drugs can also trigger violence aimed at oneself or at others. Alcoholism or drug addiction may, in addition, be an expression of an underlying neurosis or psychosis; these disorders may of themselves increase the risk of suicide. It is believed by some that any addiction, because of the incredible toll it takes on the individual both physically and emotionally, represents a form of chronic suicidal behavior.

8. Homosexuality. Homosexuals, particularly those inclined to alcoholism and depression, and those who entertain florid sadomasochistic fantasies, should be carefully assessed for suicidal potential. The ageing homosexual whose physical attractiveness is declining constitutes a serious risk. Society still continues to treat homosexuals as outcasts, thus engendering situations where homosexuals are prevented from moving within the mainstream and have to depend for support on the homosexual subculture. The homosexual subculture does not, by and large, attract persons who are noted for

their emotional stability, and so a vicious circle is established in which many homosexuals are denied exposure to stable supports. According to Socarides (1968), approximately one-half of individuals who engage in homosexual practices have concomitant schizophrenia, paranoia, are latent or pseudoneurotic schizophrenics, or are in the throes of a manic–depressive reaction. The other half, *when neurotic,* may be character disorders or addicts. Bieber *et al.* (1965), in reporting on over one hundred homosexuals who sought treatment, stated that one-third are schizophrenic, one-third are neurotic, and one-third are character disorders. While homosexuality does not necessarily denote psychopathology, it is clear that there is a high correlation and the risk of suicide is compounded.

9. Previous Suicide Attempts. Studies have shown that 50–80 per cent of those who commit suicide have a history of a previous suicide attempt (Susser, 1968).

10. Lethality of Attempt. Shneidman and Farberow (1965) divide suicides into two groups, those in which the point of no return is rapidly reached and those in which it is gradually reached. Gunshot wounds, hanging, and jumping, which are associated with a quick death, are identified almost entirely with lethal attempts, whereas wrist cutting, throat cutting, and ingestions are associated with nonfatal attempts. The more violent and painful the method chosen, the greater the risk.

The setting in which the attempt occurs (e.g., is there likelihood of immediate discovery?) and whether an attempt is made to communicate to others are important considerations. Suicidal ideas harbored by the patient and not communicated to his relatives constitute a grave situation. A suicide attempt is more serious when a note has been written. Szasz (1959) believes that suicidal behavior may constitute a form of communication, or as Shneidman and Farberow prefer, "a cry for help." A suicide attempt is less malignant when it can be determined that secondary gain is involved.

11. Living Arrangements. Suicide risk is greater among those who live alone (Susser, 1968; McMahon et al, 1963).

12. Age. Advancing age and suicide rates are directly correlated. Suicides are virtually nonexistent before nine years of age and rare in the ten to fourteen-year-old age group (less than one death for 200,000 children). However, the rate rises sharply from age fifteen to nineteen (an eight to tenfold increase); from age 20–24 the suicide rate doubles again. This trend continues to the very old adult (Shneidman and Farerow, 1957).

13. Religion. Jews and Catholics seem to have lower suicide rates than Protestants (Durkheim, 1897; Hendin, 1967).
14. Race. It appears that proportionately more blacks attempt suicide than commit it. Shneidman and Farberow report that 95% of successful suicides in their group were white. Certain subgroups are atypical; while suicide among urban black males aged 20 to 35 is nearly twice that for white men of a comparable age group, in older age groups the white suicide is significantly higher (Hendin, 1967).
15. Family History of Suicide. A history of suicide in the family must be asked about. In one series, 25% of those who attempted suicide had a history of suicide in the immediate family (Shneidman and Farberow, 1957).
16. Recent Loss. The recent loss through death of a person close to the patient has also been found to be a precipitating factor in suicide (Shneidman and Farberow, 1957).

Other factors cited as increasing the risk of suicide include hypochondriasis, recent surgery or childbirth, no apparent secondary gain, unemployment, and financial difficulty.

In evaluating a patient who has attempted suicide or is contemplating it, it is crucial to assess how depressed the patient is and to inquire specifically about guilt feelings, self-depreciation, or nihilistic ideas. The patient who persistently claims that he or others would be better off if he were dead constitutes a serious risk.

Careful attention to the above can facilitate determination of suicidal risk, but there is no conclusive way to ascertain its presence or absence. When it appears that a patient is a suicidal risk, he should then be asked how he would attempt it, whether in fact he already has a plan, how well developed the plan is, and whether the means for a serious or lethal attempt are on hand.

It is the duty of the crisis clinician to inform those around the patient as to his potential for suicide. The involvement of family or friends in his management on a crisis unit is imperative. The degree to which they are willing to become involved may well dictate the outcome of a crisis hospitalization. Where the risk of suicide is deemed serious but not grave enough to warrant confinement to a hospital, it might be necessary for family members to "special" the patient around the clock. Not only can the family actively protect the patient from his self-destructive tendencies, but they may also be able to help keep him away from situations which characteristically make him feel suicidal, e.g., the depressed patient who manifests suicidal behavior when drunk must be kept away from alcohol, at least until he has experienced a significant improvement in his mood. The enlistment of family support—and the encouragement and facilitation of *communication* between the patient and his family, so that when he feels suicidal he will turn to them—constitutes the key to the management of this patient on a crisis unit.

EVALUATION OF HOMICIDE POTENTIAL

Assessing homicidal potential may be even more difficult than assessing suicidal risk. Many people become angry and involved in fights, but few actually kill. Few studies are available of the epidemiological correlates of such behavior. Bach-Y-Rita *et al.* (1971) studied 130 patients who presented with a chief complaint of explosive violent behavior and found a high incidence of violence and alcoholism in their family histories; they themselves had often sought help for control of their violent impulses, but in vain. Their histories gave a picture of lack of control resulting in family disruption, job loss, and difficulty with the law, many having a history of arrests.

The possibility of organic factors, such as temporal lobe epilepsy, should be considered especially if the aggressive acts seem to have an episodic nature and the patient claims amnesia. An electroencephalogram may help, though not all patients with epilepsy have abnormal EEG's between seizures.

Assaultive behavior, homicidal threats, or homicide itself may be the manifestation of "displaced anger." We have seen a woman attempt to cut her daughter's throat mainly because the family had been without gas for a month. At times an assault is brought on in an overt or more often covert way by the victim; the concept of the role of victims in inviting assault suggests a new approach to violence which may prove fruitful in the management and prevention of assaultive behavior.

As with suicidal patients, alerting the relatives to the patient's destructive potential (if they do not already know) is the responsibility of the crisis worker. Naturally, the intended victim should be the first to be informed. This is one instance where the clinician should not feel constrained by issues of confidentiality. It is indefensible not to communicate to someone that his life may be in danger. Despite the patient's protests to the contrary, he is usually looking for controls, and the realization that he can talk to the therapist about murder without the latter taking the appropriate action is countertherapeutic.

Factors which might aggravate homicidal ideation, such as alcohol or drugs, should be identified, and every effort should be made to convince the patient to abstain. The institution of controls in the patient's life is essential, be it the opportunity to be seen on an emergency basis by the crisis worker or to have recourse to a priest if that helps.

Homicidal ideation of an obsessive nature is common, particularly in mothers who fear that they might harm their children. If the patient denies a conscious wish to harm the children, is very anxious about her thoughts, has good impulse control—and if there is evidence of an underlying obsessive-compulsive character disorder identifiable through undoing, reaction formation, rationalization, denial and displacement—then there is generally no need to be concerned about homicidal potential, and this should be communicated to her.

As with suicidal patients, patients who have homicidal thoughts or exhibit assaultive behavior combined with delusions and/or hallucinations must be carefully observed in a hospital, as they constitute the most serious risk.

The question of legal commitment to a mental health facility is germane to this discussion. If the clinician believes that even given the best supportive care outside the hospital that is realistically available and the ready accessibility to emergency psychiatric treatment by phone or using a 24-hour facility such as an emergency room, the patient is still a risk to himself or others because of his suicidal or homicidal impulses or behavior, it is incumbent on the clinician to have his patient certified ("committed") to a hospital for inpatient care if he does not consent to this voluntarily. State regulations vary on the circumstances of certification, but usually only one physician is needed to have the patient hospitalized for a brief period of observation. Fortunately, most patients are aware of and worried enough about their condition to agree to voluntary hospitalization.

Use of Psychotropic Agents

Most patients seen on a crisis unit do not require psychotropic medication, but those who do generally receive it early and in doses adequate to facilitate a rapid improvement. Once the diagnosis has been made that the patient is psychotic, and it has been established that there are no medical or psychiatric contraindications to the use of drugs, the appropriate medicine is prescribed in a dosage schedule aimed at effecting a rapid change in the patient's thinking, feeling, and behavior. Often all that can be hoped for is change in the patient's behavior sufficient to enable him to return to his household.

The removal of all of a psychotic patient's symptomatology is not compatible with the tasks of a crisis unit. What is necessary is to remove or reduce the symptoms which are making the patient's existence in the community intolerable to both him and to the people he is involved with at work and at home.

Schizophrenic patients usually responds rapidly to medication, be they individuals who are experiencing a first psychotic break or chronic schizophrenics in exacerbation; they can be successfully discharged within one to two weeks. Severe mood disorders generally take longer to respond to medication. Antidepressants frequently take two to three weeks to bring about a significant change in mood, and it is often necessary to refer psychotically depressed patients on for further inpatient care on an intermediate or long-term unit. By the same token, patients in the throes of a manic or hypomanic break occasionally respond to a combination of a major tranquilizer and lithium within one to two weeks, but they, too, often have to be referred on for further inpatient treatment else-where.

It is important when prescribing a drug for a psychotic to ensure that adequate provision is made for the patient to receive additional doses on a p.r.n. basis for such symptoms as restlessness, agitation, or excite-ment, and that he receive additional medication as might be necessary to guarantee him a restful sleep. This latter consideration cannot be overemphasized, and it includes the nonpsychotic patient as well. It is easy to overlook the fact that sleeping in a strange bed in unfamiliar surroundings among strangers, some of whom are psychotic, is not conducive to a good night's rest. Regardless of the diagnosis, adequate sleep both in terms of quantity and quality contribute appreciably to the removal of symptoms and to the individual's ability to accomplish objectives that are necessary for the resolution of his difficulties.

Once the patient is established on his medication the task remains to create an understanding with the patient and his family about the necessity of continuing the medication until it is mutually decided between the patient and his outpatient therapist that a reduction or cessation is in order. It frequently happens that a patient will discon-tinue the medication on his own once he feels better in an effort to convince himself that he is really not ill. Families also frequently have an intense need to deny or minimize the illness, and it is not uncommon for the parents of a young schizophrenic to talk him out of taking his medication. Another reason why this may happen is that families some-times have a conscious or unconscious investment in keeping the per-son ill. These possibilities must be kept in mind whenever the drug treatment of a psychotic patient is undertaken, and must be adequately prepared for by discussing the issues openly with the patient and his family.

The literature demonstrates that the phenothiazines and butyrophe-nones are effective in the treatment of schizophrenia, that the tricyclic antidepressants are helpful in the treatment of severe depressions, and that lithium is important in the acute and long-term management of manic–depressive illness. The psychopharmalogical agents used on a crisis unit are excellently documented in a book by Klein and Davis (1969) entitled *Diagnosis and Drug Treatment of Psychiatric Disorders.* The following is a brief description of the ones most commonly used.

1. The Phenothiazine Tranquilizers. The phenothiazine group of drugs includes a wide variety of members with varying properties such as chlorpromazine (Thorazine), thioridazine (Mellaril), per-phenazine (Trilafon), trifluoperazine (Stelazine), and fluphenazine

(Prolixin). The major psychiatric effects of the phenothiazines are behavior normalization, sleep normalization, and sedation. They are effective in controlling aggressive behavior and in reducing excitement in psychotic patients, and their use is indicated in the treatment of acute and chronic schizophrenia, agitated depressions, mania and hypomania, and some borderline states. They are also effective in reducing anxiety in a wide variety of conditions, e.g., adolescent turmoil, certain personality problems, and psychosomatic illnesses. Small doses are often effective in treating the organic psychoses. The phenothiazines are effective as sleep medications in virtually all psychiatric illnesses.

A multitude of side effects are caused by these drugs, and if a patient complains of any untoward symptom, it should be reported to a physician. The most commonly seen side effects include:

a. Dizziness with rapid changes in posture
b. Drowsiness
c. Nasal congestion
d. Dry mouth
e. Skin rashes
f. Blurred vision
g. Menstrual irregularities and lactation
h. Constipation
i. Urinary retention
j. Extrapyramidal disorders such as tremors, a Parkinson-like rigidity, and muscular spasms
k. Agranulocytosis is a serious side effect which usually manifests itself through fever and a sore throat.

Skin discoloration and pigment deposits in the eye have been described in patients receiving Thorazine or Mellaril in large doses over long periods of time.

Haloperidol (Haldol), thiothixene (Navane), and chlorprothixene (Taractan) have actions similar to those of the phenothiazines and are favored by some psychiatrists.

2. The Antidepressants.

a. The Tricyclic Antidepressants. Amitriptyline (Elavil) and imipramine (Tofranil) are frequently used on the crisis unit although they will seldom begin to affect the patient's mood during the brief stay. It is current practice to treat patients with severe depressive disorders with tricyclics, particularly where there are vegetative symptoms of depression, i.e., significant loss of weight and appetite, constipation, and a sleep disorder characterized by early morning awakening.

When it is decided to use an antidepressant, the general approach is to stabilize the patient on a schedule commensurate with his age and ability to tolerate a particular dose, and to solidify the patient's social supports such as family, friends, and supportive psychotherapy. The support of the latter helps maintain the patient during the two to three weeks it usually takes for the drug to produce an effect.

Drowsiness, dry mouth, constipation, and increased appetite are the side effects most frequently seen with the tricyclic antidepressants. 2.2 gm constitutes the average lethal dose of amitiyptyline. Great care has to be taken in prescribing these drugs, and in some situations it may be necessary to have a relative dispense the medication one tablet at a time until the patient is free of suicidal ideation. This does not hold for the phenothiazines where the incidence of reported deaths due to overdose is very low.

b. The Monoamine-Oxidase Inhibitors. Phenelzine (Nardil) and tranylcypromine (Parnate) are antidepressants that are widely used in European psychiatry but they are not used as frequently in the United States. Clinical studies have not shown them to be superior to the tricyclics, and a number of deaths have been reported due to their use or abuse. They are dangerous when taken in combination with a variety of foods, particularly those prepared by fermentation (cheese, beer, and Chianti wines) and with cold tablets, alcohol, or barbiturates.

It is believed by some, however, that there are patients who, while showing no response to tricyclic antidepressants, do respond to MAO inhibitors, and for this reason these preparations are at times prescribed. Their adverse effects, and the precautions that need to be taken, are extensively discussed in the literature, and it behooves any clinician who may be involved in the management of a patient who is receiving an MAO inhibitor to arm himself with as much information about the topic as possible.

3. Chlordiazepoxide (Librium) and Diazepam (Valium). Librium and Valium are valuable medications on a crisis unit, particularly in the treatment of withdrawal symptoms such as incipient DT's in an alcoholic. Any patient suspected of alcohol addiction is covered with Librium or Valium while on the unit.

4. Sleep Medications. Of particular value on a crisis unit are Benadryl (50–100 mg at bedtime) or Chloral hydrate (500–1000 mg at bedtime). When a patient is receiving a phenothiazine during the day, he should, however, receive additional doses of the phenothiazine if he has difficulty sleeping rather than one of these preparations.

5. Drugs for Detoxification. Due to legal restrictions barbiturates and methadone have to be obtained from sources which are legally entitled to stock them. A crisis unit has to have recourse to these sources as from time to time patients are admitted for withdrawal.

6. Lithium Carbonate. This is used as an adjunct to phenothiazines in the acute management of a manic or hypomanic episode, and in long-term prophylaxis of manic–depressive illness, where it has clearly been shown to reduce the incidence of manic or hypomanic exacerbations.

It is frequently possible on a crisis unit to reduce a manic's excitement and irritability with a phenothiazine or Haldol and then proceed with the special work-up (EKG, renal function studies) that must be obtained before starting a patient on Lithium. Thereafter he may possibly be discharged home after an additional week to two weeks on the unit; as mentioned before, however, a good number of manic or hypomanic individuals do not respond rapidly and have to be referred to a more traditional inpatient service.

7. Antiparkinson Drugs. Much controversy exists as to the advisability of routinely prescribing drugs such as benztropine mesylate (Cogentin) or procyclidine (Kemadrin) when using a phenothiazine or Haldol. While these drugs are effective in relieving the extrapyramidal side effects caused by antipsychotic agents, they cause side effects of their own, such as blurred vision and urinary retention. In addition, it is not unusual for some patients to diligently take their Cogentin while blithely forgetting or refusing to take their Trilafon. It seems reasonable, therefore, to prescribe an antiparkinson agent routinely when trifluoperazine (Stelazine), fluphenazine (Prolixin), or haloperidol (Haldol) are used, as these drugs have a high incidence of extrapyramidal side effects.

When agents such as perphenazine (Trilafon), chlorpromazine (Thorazine), or thioridazine (Mellaril) are being used, the antiparkinson agent can usually be withheld to be used only if extrapyramidal symptoms develop.

It is important to be sure that extrapyramidal side effects do not develop to the point where a patient might discontinue his medication. When antiparkinson medication does not alleviate the extrapyramidal side effects, lowering the dose of the phenothiazine may be helpful.

Only a few drugs need to be stocked on a crisis ward. Generally, it is better to know a few drugs well and to use these when indicated rather than to experiment with many different drugs. Of course, this concept applies to all of medicine, but it has particular relevance to a crisis unit where so much depends on what can be accomplished in a few days.

The Stay on the Crisis Unit

Pragmatism in determining the duration of the stay should be the characteristic of a crisis unit. Different patients with the same diagnosis may have widely varying needs depending upon their social network outside the hospital, their response to medication, and their ability to utilize an outpatient disposition. Length of stay may vary from one day to two weeks. If it is felt that a patient may require more than two weeks to pull together, one must seriously query whether admission to a crisis unit is appropriate in the first place. If a referring clinician tells an admitting staff member that hospitalizations have generally lasted several months for a given patient, it might be advisable to recommend referral to a longer-term unit directly. Unfortunately, there is no definitive way to predict the duration of stay, and if there seems to be even a remote possibility of discharge within ten to fourteen days the patient should be given the benefit of the doubt.

The general thrust should be toward rapid discharge, and often it is advantageous to ask a patient at the time of admission or soon thereafter how long he predicts he will require before he feels ready for discharge. If the answer is reasonable an attempt should be made to achieve that goal. However, while rapid discharge should be the predominant ethic, if a patient is likely to do better if given a few extra days to stabilize on medication and to organize a more solid living arrangement, the time should be granted. Thus, pragmatism rather than rigid formulas should be the guiding principle.

Due to the rapid turnover there are often patients on the unit at a particular time who are at different phases of hospitalization. On one hand this encourages patients by allowing them to see that discharge is indeed possible despite what to them seems like an horrendous psychic state; on the other hand, they may get the "discharge jitters" when newly made friends are discharged before them. This phenomenon should be explained so that the patient can continue to work at a pace consistent with his own abilities towards his own discharge.

The tasks to be accomplished by the crisis teams during the hospitalization, depending on the patient, are as follows:

1. Completion of the Evaluation. This includes not only the history, mental status examination, physical examination with indicated laboratory tests, but also observation of the patient's behavior on the ward. Therefore, basic nursing skills are needed in observing and recording how a patient eats, sleeps, and interacts with others, including visiting family and friends. Depending on the patient, this part of the evaluation may take one or several days.

2. Clarification of the Problems Bringing the Patient to the Hospital. Sometimes this may be accomplished quickly as a patient may clearly state these at the time of admission, e.g., a patient with a severe grief reaction. In other cases, as in a severely acting out promiscuous adolescent, it may take several sessions of family evaluation to assess difficulties, such as an affair a parent is having, which may have contributed to the patient's behavioral change. In still others there may be no clear-cut precipitant even after a systematic search has been made, and here stabilization on medication may be all that is required.

3. Communication of Important Decisions to Significant People. The staff should aid a patient in communicating decisions arrived at while on the unit to those whom the decisions affect. This includes decisions arrived at prior to admission. In the latter case, guilt or external circumstances may have prevented the patient from verbalizing the decisions, or if he did, it was only at great cost to his social or psychic equilibrium. Such decisions as quitting school, separation from a spouse, terminating relationships, or negotiating an abortion are difficult to communicate at times, and may require the assistance and support of the staff.

4. Involvement in Outpatient Therapy. As stated earlier, for patients with long-term problems, brief follow-up therapy may not be sufficient and the task of the crisis team may be to decide with the patient on an appropriate plan for outpatient treatment. In such a

case, the crisis hospitalization is seen as the initial phase in a long course of treatment.

5. Resolution of Incapacitating Symptomatology. For psychotic patients the duration of hospitalization is determined primarily by the length of time required for resolution of the symptoms to a level which will permit him to function outside the hospital. If, on admission, he has a viable living arrangement, he will need little other therapeutic input other than brief contact, medication, periodic evaluation, and the inherent structure of the ward.

6. Reduction or Resolution of Suicidal or Homicidal Ideation. The word *reduction* is used because it is not uncommon that some patients may remain chronically suicidal. The task of the unit is then to reduce the immediacy of such thinking so that the patient can continue treatment out of the hospital. Such individuals may require continuous or intermittent follow-up treatment for the remainder of their lives. These patients should be told that the unit will continue to be available when destructive impulses begin to become overwhelming and that they need only present themselves to the outpatient department or the emergency room to receive attention to their problems. On the other hand, there are individuals in whom complete resolution of suicidal ideation is accomplished during a crisis hospitalization.

7. Completion of Detoxification. Patients admitted to our unit for detoxification are usually already being followed elsewhere, and the major task of the unit is merely to withdraw the patient from drugs or alcohol.

8. Acceptance of the Realities of the Situation. Some suicidal patients, particularly those who are admitted following ingestions, maintain the fantasy that prompted the attempt, e.g., that a lover will return. Others, more seriously ill, may be admitted at the behest of family members who have a vague, ill-defined hope that the patient's behavior will somehow miraculously be changed. In both instances the expectations of the patient or his family must be identified and adjusted so that the patient may function with less intrusion from feelings derived from unrealistic expectations. It is important that the staff not collude in the unrealistic hopes because of their own intrapsychic needs or rescue fantasies. It is helpful to outline to the patient and his family from the beginning what can and what cannot be changed.

9. Acceptance of Structure and Medication. Psychiatric patients, especially schizophrenics, often present because of insufficient

structure in their lives or because of a need for medication which they should have been taking. While the patient's and his relatives' ambivalent desires for him to remain sick play a role which cannot be changed in a brief period, one must appeal to the healthy aspects of both to order the patient's existence and help him to remain on medication. This may require daily sessions with the patient and the family reviewing the reality of the outcome if the recommendations are not followed, and the events preceding the present confinement which were due to his not adhering to essential treatment.

10. Finding Employment. While it may not always be possible for unemployed patients to find a job while on the unit, if search is begun, a significant number will later be successful. Regular working hours impose structure in a person's life, and the return to work makes a significant contribution to one's self-esteem and economic security. The lack of any of these three factors is a frequent precipitant leading to hospitalization on a crisis unit.

11. Readjustment of the Family System. For some patients with severe characterological problems or chronic psychotic states, adjustment of the familial equilibrium may be important. A series of family meetings initially for evaluation and subsequently to affect a therapeutic intervention is needed. Eventual discharge may depend on the acceptance by the family of outpatient family therapy.

12. Arranging an Appropriate Disposition. This, unfortunately, is not always as easy as it may seem and all the help the staff can obtain from family and friends of the patient may be required. Innovative and pragmatic dispositions are required, as will be taken up in the next chapter.

Episodic hospitalization may be needed for some chronically ill patients. The fact that this occurs should not be interpreted to the patient or family as disastrous. Rather, for patients whose alternative is public hospital confinements lasting years, *episodic hospitalization* is a likely occurrence and is in no sense a failure. Such readmissions for chronic patients, if they last only a matter of days, are a success in that they prevent the debilitating effects of chronic institutionalization and afford such individuals a measure of self-esteem and comfort.

Disposition of Patients

Patients who present with a traditional crisis such as a grief reaction may need only a course of brief outpatient psychotherapy such as can often be provided by a member of the crisis team. Others, such as those undergoing an acute psychotic decompensation, are just beginning a prolonged course of treatment, and the hospitalization represents a stage during which assessment is performed, treatment is *instituted*, and plans are made for long-term follow-up.

In most cases, it is the task of the crisis unit to effect remission or reduction of symptoms so that outpatient treatment can begin. Selection of the appropriate follow-up and helping the patient—and in some situations his family—to accept it, constitute integral and important aspects of crisis hospitalization.

The disposition of patients from any inpatient facility presents problems. Lack of motivation on the part of patients, their need to deny their illness, and sabotage of treatment plans by family members are typical problems that are encountered.

Due to the rapid turnover of patients on a crisis unit, additional factors come into play. In many communities there is a dearth of the facilities needed to absorb large numbers of patients, some of whom are in need of specialized services, e.g., methadone maintenance programs, vocational rehabilitation centers, branches of gamblers anonymous. This is magnified if the crisis staff lacks familiarity with those services that are available.

In addition, errors in clinical judgment regarding disposition are much more likely to occur where there is a rapid turnover of patients and where the staff is provided with but a day or two in which to evaluate the patient and his family.

These problems can be minimized if:

1. Adequate resources for referrals are or can be made available in a community
2. The crisis staff, through the medium of seminars and visits, becomes familiar with those services that do exist
3. A pragmatic approach to disposition is used
4. The staff is disposition-oriented so that evaluation of a patient's ultimate disposition commences when he is admitted
5. The unit has a 30-day follow-up outpatient program. Not only can this provide definitive treatment for numerous patients, but it allows for assessment to continue for those patients whose ultimate disposition is uncertain; this applies particularly to referrals for couples therapy and family therapy. The pattern of a couple's or of a family's interaction changes somewhat when a member is hospitalized. Spouses or families may defer to the judgment of a clinician while the patient is in the hospital but following discharge changes in motivation occur and commitments made while the patient is in the hospital may be broken. When, for instance, couples therapy has been agreed upon and a spouse later refuses to attend couple's meetings, the situation can be salvaged by referring the patient to another form of treatment.

THE EVALUATION OF PATIENTS FOR REFERRAL

The first decision that has to be made is whether a patient needs further inpatient treatment beyond that which the unit can provide. If inpatient treatment is not indicated, the next determination is whether the patient requires outpatient treatment. There are some situations (e.g., the melodrama) where outpatient treatment may not be necessary and, in fact, may be contraindicated. Most patients admitted to the crisis unit, however, do require follow-up.

Once it has been decided that outpatient treatment is indicated, the next step is to determine what kind of treatment. The choice here lies between psychotherapy—individual, family, or group therapy—or a program such as Alcoholics Anonymous, a medication maintenance program, or school counseling.

THE SELECTION OF PATIENTS FOR PSYCHOTHERAPY

The criteria for deciding whether a patient is suitable for psychodynamic psychotherapy include:

1. Motivation for treatment
2. The ability to persevere
3. A stable life situation in terms of domestic environment and work situation
4. An adequate intellectual endowment and capacity for introspection
5. Reasonable acquaintance with the English language. (There are, however, institutions where therapists conduct individual or group therapy in languages other than English, e.g., Spanish, Italian, and Eastern European languages.)
6. The ability to tolerate the pain, anxiety, anger, and other feelings that come to the surface during therapy
7. The capacity to talk about feelings rather than "act out"
8. The capacity to accept one's own role in creating the problems one is confronted with, rather than habitually blaming others

The forms of psychotherapy are:

1. Brief Psychotherapy. This usually consists of ten to twelve 50-minute interviews which focus on the current life difficulties, rather than attempting to explore the past in depth. It is most suitable for a person who has become symptomatic around a specific crisis, e.g., loss of a dear one, promotion, graduation, marriage or divorce.
2. Long-term Psychotherapy. This consists of from one to three, 50-minute interviews per week, and varies in duration from months to many years. This form of treatment is generally indicated for the neuroses, nonorganic psychoses, personality disturbances, and psychophysiological disorders.
3. Group Therapy. Groups consist of from six to ten patients who meet with a single therapist or two cotherapists for a 90-minute session once or sometimes twice a week. The duration varies from brief treatment (ten to twelve sessions) to a year or years. Group therapy has many applications but is most appropriate for the following patients:

a. The socially withdrawn, shy person who has difficulty asserting himself

b. Those who have severe conflicts around their relationships with authority figures

c. Adolescents with a wide variety of diagnoses, e.g., schizophrenia, borderline states, adjustment reactions, sexual problems

d. Patients whose characterological makeup makes it difficult for them to get along with others

e. Patients who cannot relate to an individual therapist without becoming overly dependent, or who characteristically "act out" around a dyadic relationship with a therapist

4. Specialized Groups. Group therapy has been successfully employed in the treatment of alcoholics, drug addicts, and patients with psychophysiological disorders such as asthma. New applications of group therapy are continually evolving. These include behavior group therapy for patients with incapacitating phobias, for obese patients, and for patients with hysterical disorders; group therapy for mothers who experience serious difficulties in raising their children; and couples groups. Where severe marital disharmony exists this approach provides a forum where couples can share difficulties and positive experiences, discover that their problems are not unique, and learn from others who "have been through it all" healthy ways of coping with the demands of marriage and child rearing.

Family group therapy allows families to share experiences, provide support and encouragement to each other, and to suggest more adaptive ways of coping to each other.

5. Medication, Support, and Rehabilitation Groups. These groups do not emphasize psychotherapy and do not require that participants in any way be candidates for psychotherapy. A patient is required simply to attend regularly and behave himself in a reasonably appropriate manner.

The provision of these groups by outpatient departments has been found to contribute significantly to maintaining chronically disturbed patients in the community. Their task is to provide support, rehabilitation, and medication—either one or a combination of these. Many who have drifted repeatedly through various inpatient facilities and outpatient psychotherapies become stabilized by these groups, where warmth, respect, and support are provided, usually along with psychotropic medications. They constitute in many instances the follow-up that is best suited to patients seen on the crisis unit.

REFERRALS MADE FROM A CRISIS UNIT

1. Brief Outpatient Treatment by Crisis Unit Staff. This is generally limited to four to six weeks and is reserved for patients who are fairly well integrated; patients whose crisis can be expected to resolve rapidly; patients awaiting referral, e.g., to a therapy group; couples and families needing evaluation to determine the appropriateness of a referral to couples therapy or family therapy. Occasionally, longer-term outpatient therapy contracts are undertaken by members of the crisis team. This should be encouraged only if it does not interfere with the primary responsibility, namely, inpatient crisis patients.

2. Outpatient Private Therapy. In the case of a decision for private therapy it is necessary to determine whether the patient has the funds to pay for it and if he is willing to do so. An evaluation should take into account what health insurance coverage the patient has. It is generally preferable to refer patients to private therapists rather than to clinics for these reasons: Public clinics are often overloaded and should be reserved for patients who clearly cannot afford private treatment; also the continuous staff turnover in training settings is a disadvantage to patients because it interrupts the continuity of care. Continuity can be more easily maintained in private settings. Private therapists include psychiatrists, psychoanalytic-psychiatrists, psychologists, social workers, and counselors. The fees vary according to the area as well as to the training of the therapist. The cost of group therapy is significantly lower than that for individual therapy.

3. Outpatient Treatment Programs Within the Center. Referral to outpatient follow-up can be expedited when outpatient facilities exist in the center that houses the crisis unit. The facilities that are most useful are a medication support and rehabilitation unit, a group therapy unit, and an individual psychotherapy unit.

4. Drug and A.A. Programs. Alcoholics Anonymous will often go out of its way to facilitate the referral process. Drug programs vary in how aggressively they seek people for treatment. Organizations such as Daytop and Synanon operate residential drug treatment programs in many communities. In either case, contacts with such

agencies should be initiated while patients are in the hospital. Often patients can begin to attend A.A. meetings while they are still inpatients.

5. Adolescent Treatment Programs. Many communities are now developing "crash-pad" treatment centers for youths with difficulties. These centers frequently refer those whom they feel cannot be properly managed outside a hospital to the crisis unit; they also take back patients for follow-up care. It is important that good communication with the staff of youth programs be maintained because of their inherent distrust of "establishment" institutions such as mental health centers. It is important that they understand what services the crisis unit can provide and how their clients might be able to use such assistance. If mutual understanding is fostered, it is likely to result in young patients availing themselves of services they would otherwise not seek except under duress. Thus, the endorsement by the crisis staff of the services provided by trusted youth centers is valuable in terms of patient care.

6. Relatives. Occasions arise where the provision of a protective, stable environment can benefit a patient more than a referral for psychotherapy. An obvious example would be an adolescent whose home life is chaotic and whose time on the unit represents an effort to involve her parents in psychiatric treatment. If the evaluation reveals that the home situation is indeed intolerable and that the patient does not have a significant psychiatric disturbance, then disposition should be geared toward finding a stable living arrangement, such as the home of a relative who is concerned about the patient and is prepared to take over parental responsibilities. Such an arrangement would not preclude the initiation of psychiatric treatment (such as an adolescent group) if it were indicated but would constitute the major thrust in terms of disposition.

7. School Counselors and Social Workers. Adolescents are frequently referred by counselors for evaluation because of difficulties in their school performance. Assessment may reveal that intellectual endowment is limited or that there is evidence of minimal neurological impairment. In such an instance formal psychiatric treatment might not be as valuable as would the making of alterations in the school program. In fact, unless there are specific indications that psychiatric therapy is likely to be helpful, it should be avoided lest the patient have then to deal with the dual burden of intellectual and psychological impairment. When a referral is made to school officials, they can be assisted in restructuring the student's program

as well as in offering support within the context of the school. Continuing consultation for the officials related to the area of the problems should be made available.

8. Nonpsychiatric Physicians or Clinics. Some patients may require only continuing medication following evaluation and brief treatment on a crisis unit. Their problems may be primarily medical (e.g., hypothyroidism) or they may feel that they are able to benefit more from contact with their usual family physician. Such patients may quite appropriately be referred to their clinics or physicians. Referral should be made while the patient is hospitalized and the willingness of the physician to prescribe psychotropic medications on an ongoing basis can be ascertained. Often willingness is enhanced if continuing consultation is offered and if immediate guidelines such as dosage of medication and length of treatment are suggested.

9. The Clergy and Church Groups. Patients may be appropriately referred to clergy and church groups following discharge from the hospital in cases where they have had precrisis interest and involvement with the church. This may be particularly helpful for isolated patients, those who have limited confidence in psychiatry, and those who have strong faith in the church.

10. Inpatient Treatment at a Public Hospital. Not all patients seen on a crisis unit will be able to reconstitute in the brief time available. When this is not possible, and in the absence of financial resources or insurance coverage for private hospitalization, the patient must be transferred to a public psychiatric hospital where the time and structure necessary for further rehabilitation and stabilization can be provided. It is no secret that staffing and funding are limited in most of these institutions. For most patients this does not retard recovery in that the natural course of the illness when treated with medication is not altered by the setting. What is of more significance regarding such institutions is that patients are forced to be away from their home communities, and as a result their follow-up care is not carefully worked out.

11. Inpatient Treatment in Private Facilities. For patients with financial resources who require longer hospitalization, private inpatient treatment facilities provide valuable service. Generally, the range of services at private centers is greater than at public hospitals, and efforts should be made to use them. Also, public hospitals tend to be overcrowded and understaffed and often located at considerable distances from people's homes, thus creating hardships for the en-

tire family. In making referrals to private hospitals, one should be familiar with all the hospitals in the area so that the best possible referral can be made.

12. School and Work Clinics. Many large industries and schools—especially universities—have clinics for the care of employees and students. These provide a range of services, and frequently patients can obtain aftercare in these settings.

13. Halfway Houses. Patients with insurmountable difficulties at home, those who lack a stable living arrangement, and patients with certain kinds of psychopathology (e.g., borderline states) can benefit from living in a halfway house. These are usually supervised by people with some psychological expertise, and the structured living situation can be quite helpful and work against regression. Patients often make the necessary arrangements while in the hospital and move to a halfway house when discharged.

14. Communes. This unconventional disposition is often overlooked because of its lack of psychiatric affiliation. However, communes can provide a unique type of group support for individuals without other living arrangements. Patients who are more deeply disturbed are likely to fare better in halfway houses.

15. Family Agencies. Many crisis patients require family or couple's treatment over a protracted period following discharge. Referral might be made to any of a variety of agencies providing such services. Because the agencies often have religious or ethnic affiliations, patients' preferences should be considered in arranging such a disposition.

16. Nursing or Convalescent Homes. Senile patients are sometimes admitted to a crisis unit when their families are no longer able to care for them. If the patient's behavior is not mitigated by a trial of medication, referral to a convalescent home may be necessary. The choice of one rests on these considerations: what the patient and his family can afford; the services that are provided, e.g., it is advantageous if the facility has good medical care; the location—continuing contact with the family is facilitated if the convalescent home is situated within a reasonable distance.

18. Medical Inpatient Facilities. Sometimes a neuropsychiatric evaluation reveals that the patient requires immediate medical treatment. For instance, disturbed behavior may be secondary to an organic brain syndrome which is the result of a cerebrovascular episode. In such a case immediate transfer should be arranged to a general hospital where the patient can receive intensive medical care.

19. Other Community Agencies. Among the patients admitted to a crisis unit, some have particular problems for which nonpsychiatric agencies can offer assistance. The Welfare Department, The Division of Vocational Rehabilitation, Welfare Moms, Woman's Liberation, Gay Liberation, and Legal Assistance fall under this rubric. In general, these organizations deal with extrapsychic needs and problems such as poverty, discrimination, and legal aid. Referral to them may be helpful in reducing stress for some patients.

20. Ethnic Organizations. Much has been written about the detrimental effects of rapid cultural shifts. Subgroups in the United States such as the Spanish-speaking Puerto Rican populations in some of the large urban areas reflect these problems. Patients with such backgrounds sometimes come in overwhelmed by an alien and, at times, overtly hostile environment. A Spanish community organization can be an appropriate disposition for such patients.

21. No Referral. Patients occasionally do not need referral, or are unresponsive to suggestions for further treatment, or both. An example would be a mildly histrionic female who ingests a few pain tablets to get her errant boyfriend to return to her, and who openly acknowledges the manipulative nature of her actions. Following a tearful reunion with the boyfriend on the unit she might state that she no longer is in need of help; this may well be an accurate perception.

22. Referral Back to Therapy. Many patients admitted to a crisis unit are already in outpatient treatment. Once the reasons for the admission have been clarified and communicated between the parties involved (patient, staff, and outpatient clinician), the patient will usually be referred back to his therapist for continuing treatment.

The dispositions described are not mutually exclusive but may be combined to maximize a patient's chances for survival in the community. For a separated, unemployed mother of seven children who comes in because of depression a brief treatment program, with the institution of antidepressants, may be combined with collaboration with welfare workers and a homemaker agency.

Every referral should be made personally by a clinician who has worked with the patient. A "hand-carried" referral facilitates the communication of information both to an agency and from an agency to the unit, and indirectly to the patient. This enables all staff members to learn about the resources available for patients, and conveys information about the unit to those agencies likely to have occasion to refer patients to the unit.

Discharge summaries should be dictated promptly on all patients discharged. When appropriate, a copy should be sent to the clinician assuming continuing care for the patient and a copy entered in the patient's ongoing record at the center. Finally, a copy should be sent to the referring clinician, particularly when the patient was admitted for evaluation.

ILLUSTRATIVE EXAMPLES OF CRISIS INTERVENTION

The Psychotic Patient

THE MANIC PATIENT

Perhaps the most interesting psychiatric presentation, though one of the most difficult to manage, is the person in the manic phase of manic–depressive illness. He or she may present as a confident, ebullient extrovert who seems to have boundless energy and often a charming affability. Manic patients can be very difficult to control, however, when their excitement and aggressive self-assertiveness boil over. Prompt and vigorous use of pharmacologic agents if combined with firmness, tact, and patience can bring the symptoms under control within days. The clinician's output of energy and time in the treatment of this illness may well be rewarded, as these patients tend to be able to function between their psychotic episodes.

The advent of the use of lithium carbonate has dramatically altered the course of this disease, by reducing symptoms during the acute phase and by reducing the frequency of manic exacerbations. Lithium carbonate used to be restricted but it can be safely administered now wherever laboratories are available for the serial estimation of serum levels.

CASE HISTORY

M. P., a 32-year-old, white, Protestant, married father of two children, was admitted from the emergency room where his wife and three neighbors had taken him after he had told her he intended to buy an expensive sports car and drive to the West Coast to close a business deal; the patient was a salesman for a small electronics firm. Ten days prior to admission he had begun to talk animatedly about "a tremendous opportunity for expansion" that only he could negotiate. He told his wife that the consummation of the deal would bring in millions and that he would be able to retire within a few years. He began to stay up all night making elaborate plans for what he intended to do with his riches and reacted to his wife's questions with scorn, jocularity, and occasional outbursts of abusiveness. Mrs. P. recognized that he was in the midst of an exacerbation but was unable to persuade him to go to the emergency room. She was eventually able to enlist the aid of neighbors to bring her husband in for treatment.

On the ward the patient was restless, excitable, and argumentative. This combined with his rapid shifts in thought, made history-taking impossible. His wife, however, was able to provide information. Mr. P., the youngest of three children, was from a small town in the Midwest. His childhood was apparently normal but when he reached adolescence he became somewhat moody. He attended college in a city near his hometown and was elected president of his class after serving for a year as social chairman for his fraternity. During his senior year he started dating his present wife, and following graduation they married and moved to the East Coast, where he felt his opportunities would be better. As a salesman for the electronics firm, he was a steady but not spectacular worker. He responded very positively to the birth of a son and a daughter and was a devoted father.

Three years prior to the current hospitalization, Mr. P. was admitted to a private psychiatric facility following the sudden onset, without obvious precipitant, of a manic episode. He was hospitalized at that time for three months and given phenothiazines and electroshock treatment. Upon discharge he refused outpatient referral, and remained free of significant symptomatology for three years. His performance at work, however, vacillated from months when he was the top salesman to others when he seemed "down" and was unable to sell anything. His family history was significant in that his paternal grandfather and a paternal aunt both had periodic depressions requiring hospitalization.

On the ward the patient was excited, easily overstimulated and irritable; he was totally sleepless the first night despite adequate doses of haloperidol. He was extremely disruptive to the ward partly because the other patients were fascinated by his infectious enthusiasm. The day following admission a medical evaluation for lithium was performed (EKG, serum electrolytes, serum creatinine, blood urea nitrogen, and a urinalysis), and within 48 hours of his admission lithium carbonate therapy was instituted in addition to the haloperidol. The lithium was raised by daily increments to 2.4 gm/day. By the sixth day he began to sleep more than six hours a night, and his grandiose delusions began to dissolve. He gradually regained a normal mood and by the twelfth day was ready for discharge. Interviews with him and joint meetings with his wife failed to reveal any obvious stress in his recent life to account for the manic break. Both were impressed by the rapid clearing of his symptoms and agreed with the staff that he should remain on lithium indefinitely.

Mr P. called his employer and his return to work was arranged without any difficulty. He was discharged home to be followed by a nearby clinic which specializes in the administration of lithium to outpatients.

Patients with manic–depressive illness are often free of the major social deterioration characteristic of schizophrenia. It is thus of major value to maintain their social adaptation by attempting to treat them without sending them out of the community to state hospitals. This requires experience with lithium and the ability to handle the patient skillfully while he is on the ward. It is often necessary to make certain adjustments when such patients are on the unit. They should not be overstimulated and should be allowed to remain out of meetings or alone, if necessary, when they are in an excited phase. The usual gathering of information, social assessments, and interventions characteristic of crisis treatment should be postponed until the patient is able to tolerate them.

THE ACUTE SCHIZOPHRENIC

The diagnosis of schizophrenia should be considered when any moderately disturbed young person presents for psychiatric treatment. Unfortunately, unless flagrant cognitive and perceptual disturbances are present, the presence of schizophrenia may be missed. It is, therefore, all the more important that a careful longitudinal psychosocial history be taken in addition to close observation of the patient's mental status over the course of a few days. Intoxicants such as alcohol or the hallucinogens may mask the symptoms and may in fact have been taken by the patient in an attempt to deal with his deteriorating mental condition. Frequently, once the diagnosis has been made and the appropriate psychotropic drug treatment commenced a patient may be able to return to the community soon, as the following case illustrates.

CASE HISTORY

A. S., a 22-year-old, white, divorced woman, was admitted to the crisis unit from the emergency room with the diagnosis of "hysterical personality." One year prior to admission—at the time of the break-up of the patient's marriage, which had lasted but three weeks—the patient began to undergo marked social deterioration, though she continued to function adequately at her job as a secretary. She became promiscuous, was unable to maintain residence at any place for more than one month, and became peripherally involved with the hippie subculture. She had occasionally visited her parents who lived in the area but would not stay with them more than a day at a time. Eventually, she began to experience pressure at work; she told her mother, "My head is splitting apart and I need help." Then her parents brought her to the emergency room.

On the unit she presented as an attractive woman who behaved in a flirtatious and seductive manner. She told us in a coquettish way that she wanted the staff to help her get her head back together. On the initial mental status examination she was somewhat vague, but seemed to be without a thought or perceptual disorder. Her recent functioning was, however, suggestive of schizophrenia and so a series of mental status examinations were planned along with careful observation of her behavior on the ward.

When the mental status examination was repeated the following day, she exhibited blocking, circumstantiality, and hypervigilance, and told the interviewer that she now trusted the staff sufficiently to reveal that she frequently heard voices calling her a whore.

She was begun on phenothiazines and within four days seemed considerably more comfortable. She now stated that she no longer heard voices and that her thinking was clearer than it had been for a year, since in fact, the time she had decided to get married.

The patient was able to communicate better with her parents in joint meetings and clearly expressed her wish to move back home and cease her unfulfilling acting-out behavior. Her parents agreed to this proposed disposition, and she was discharged to outpatient follow-up.

This case illustrates the use of the longitudinal psychosocial case history as an ancillary diagnostic tool on a crisis unit. It is especially useful if one is attempting to diagnose an illness like schizophrenia when accurate diagnosis can lead to the initiation of the appropriate pharmacological treatment and minimize the occurence of frequent rehospitalization because of misdiagnosis. The value of a short-term crisis ward for observing changes in the patient's mental status and behavior is demonstrated. Often a synthesis of information from multiple sources e.g., psychosocial history, mental status examination, and physical examination—and observation of a patient's response to a trial of medication—is necessary before a valid diagnosis can be made.

The rapid response of this patient to phenothiazines is typical of schizophrenic patients treated on a crisis unit. This suggests that many schizophrenics, especially first-break schizophrenics, should be afforded the opportunity to recompensate on a short-term crisis unit rather than being referred ab initio to long-term units. The supportive structure of a well-staffed unit and vigorous use of medication can splint a disintegrating ego during the height of the illness.

Without the use of psychopharmacological agents in doses sufficient to control the patient's disruptive behavior, schizophrenics cannot be treated on a crisis unit. Contrary to what has traditionally been taught, the immediate use of psychotropic agents may *facilitate* the task of evaluation, allowing the planning for a patient's disposition to begin early in the hospitalization.

The atmosphere on a crisis unit is in fact conducive to the rapid resolution of acute schizophrenic symptomatology. The short stay that is allotted to patients, the problem-solving orientation of the staff, the rapid flow of other patients through the unit, and the general tone of optimism for an early discharge all help to undercut regression. Most acute schizophrenics can be discharged within a week to ten days, not only free of the psychotic symptoms that interfere, but with some gains having been made in terms of work, home, and school.

THE CHRONIC SCHIZOPHRENIC

The chronic schizophrenic usually presents around a disruption in his life such as the vacation of his or her therapist, a loss in the family, stress around a maturational problem, or cessation of medication. Sometimes a careful search for a precipitating event will be unrewarding, and in these cases attention should be focused on attempting to achieve symptomatic improvement and reintegrate the patient into his social milieu.

At times one's evaluation leaves one with the impression that either the patient, his family, or both want a "rest." The healing effects of a few days in a protective, structured, and supportive setting in the life of a chronic schizophrenic should not be belittled. Some adjustment in the patient's social or work situations can be made, but attempts to effect intrapsychic change generally prove to be fruitless.

CASE HISTORY

C. S., an attractive, 40-year-old, black divorcee with a history of many previous psychiatric hospitalizations in excess of two months, was admitted through the emergency room, where she had been taken because of hallucinations, delusions of grandeur, and restlessness. She was somewhat incoherent and perseverated, answering every question with the word "true."

We learned from the patient's oldest daughter that the patient's mother had died the previous afternoon from a massive upper gastrointestinal hemorrhage. Upon returning from the hospital, Mrs. S. informed her family that she didn't have the strength to attend the funeral. After this, she was observed by the family to become increasingly upset and began to "talk crazy."

Mrs. S.'s excited psychotic behavior was rapidly brought under control with a phenothiazine and she was subsequently encouraged to discuss her feelings about her mother's death and her inability to attend the funeral, but no attempt was made to focus on this. Rather, she was supported in her decision not to attend.

The day following the funeral all evidence of psychotic thinking and behavior disappeared. It was our impression that the patient had retreated into psychosis in order to avoid a stressful situation, as she also had in the past. This view was supported by the dramatic remission of the psychotic symptoms following the funeral.

During the course of the brief hospitalization, we learned that Mrs. S. had been having difficulty coping with the demands of her six children, and we therefore helped her to obtain the assistance of a homemaker through the State Welfare office. This accomplished, she was discharged to a supportive group in a medication clinic.

Clearly, no effort was made (nor do we believe is possible to be made) in curing this patient's chronic schizophrenia. It is likely that she was chronically psychotic but not in a manner which was evident to others. A conscientious effort was therefore made to ameliorate her symptomatology with medication and to investigate only the factors precipitating the present admission and decompensation. As a result, she was able to return home within a few days in contrast to her usual course of many weeks.

If a crisis mode of treatment is employed with some of the most profound or chronic psychiatric illnesses, many patients can return home to their preexisting level of functioning in a relatively short period of time. We feel that this type of approach is justified given the lack of impressive evidence from the use of more intensive and long-term treatment of these conditions. For patients with chronic schizophrenia, a willingness to continue taking phenothiazines and to exist at home even at a marginal level of adjustment is usually preferable to life-long institutionalization, with its insidious deterioration of social adjustment.

THE INVOLUTIONAL PSYCHOTIC

Involutional psychosis often presents as a combination of depressive and paranoid symptoms although purer states, especially of depression, are encountered. Because such patients are generally in their fifties or sixties, organic pathology must always be ruled out; combinations of such with a psychogenic psychosis are often encountered. A certain amount of paranoid ideation, in addition to memory loss, may be a frequent concomitant of the aging process. It is imperative to remember that the incidence of suicide increases with age (Shneidman and Farberow, 1957).

While many involutional patients require several weeks of hospitalization, some respond rapidly to the supportive structure of a crisis unit, as the following case illustrates.

CASE HISTORY

I. P. is a 51-year-old, university trained, unmarried engineer employed in a large industry. He was brought to the emergency room by his brother after telling him that he had "crazy thoughts" and that he wanted to talk to a psychiatrist.

Three weeks prior to his admission to the crisis unit, two vice-presidents in the firm had been asked to resign due to severe financial cutbacks. A few days after this, the patient had begun to feel that different colors had different meanings for him: "Everyone at work would wear yellow one day and red the next." He was convinced that his co-workers were plotting to interfere with his work, and he therefore stayed in his laboratory until late at night, as he said, "until everyone had left to go home." When he eventually went home at night he slept very little and would lie in his bed thinking, "If I lose my job, they'll send me back."

The patient emigrated to the United States from an Eastern European country after the end of World War II. Skilled in his field, he found employment easily, and at the time of his admission was still working for the company he had joined in 1948. He never really assimilated himself into the pluralistic American society but identified strongly with others of his ethnic background. He belonged to a number of societies and clubs whose membership was confined to his ethnic group, and he was also a devout member of his national church.

Mr. P. led a rather seclusive life but enjoyed the clubs and attended his church regularly. He drank occasionally and once or twice a year became drunk over a weekend; he could not be deemed an alcoholic. Save for a married brother who lived nearby, his entire family perished during the war.

The patient presented as a distinguished-looking, quiet-spoken middle-aged man who was fully oriented and was without evidence of an organic brain syndrome. A clear history of ideas of reference and persecutory delusions was elicited, but there was no evidence of a thought disorder or of hallucinations. He had retained insight into his symptomatology and told us, with a smile, that he would like us to give him some medicine that would help his crazy thoughts diminish. The diagnosis was made of an involutional paranoid state and a treatment program of phenothiazines and therapeutic interviewing was begun together with a search for resources.

During interviews Mr. P. reported that after the vice-presidents were fired, he had become afraid of his own position. Since he was in this country as a resident alien, he might be considered "of no value to America" and be recalled to his native country in Eastern Europe. As his psychosis cleared he was able to tell us that his preoccupation with colors was a symbolic reflection of his mixed allegiance to the American flag, his native country, and the red flag of the U.S.S.R., which had invaded his country at the end of the war. We also learned that for years he had been a staunch supporter of his church but that his interest had declined after the church had moved. With the help of the patient's brother we were able to locate a comparable church as well as a club of people from their country in a nearby city. The patient was discharged after a five-day hospitalization to a private therapist.

This case illustrates that some patients with involutional psychosis do, in fact, respond to treatment quite rapidly. Even when this is the case, it is important to make sure that they are well supervised in the immediate post-hospitalization period inasmuch as single male patients in Mr. P.'s age group represent the highest suicide risks.

Of note regarding this patient is that his treatment was geared entirely to his symptoms and his social system. The use of medications and the implementation of minor adjustments in his social network made him considerably more comfortable and less lonely. He was encouraged to use his social resources to their fullest extent as a means of avoiding the conditions which contributed to his crisis.

THE PATIENT WITH A DRUG PSYCHOSIS

With the prevalence of hallucinogenic drug use in the general population, especially by adolescents and young adults, crisis units are frequently called upon to treat and assess people who present with drug reactions. Amphetamines, marijuana, and lysergic acid diethylamide (LSD) are the most commonly involved substances. Unquestionably, there is concern among youth about contact with "establishment" institutions such as psychiatric treatment centers, and so those who do come tend to have serious intoxications and reactions. Many others are protected by friends or less formal treatment centers in the community through the course of the reaction.

The approach of a crisis unit is twofold: 1) to treat the acute intoxication; 2) to assess, as with other patients, the presence of premorbid psychopathology and arrange for treatment, as the following case demonstrates.

CASE HISTORY

D.P. is a 20-year-old, white, single female who was admitted from the emergency room with the diagnosis of a drug reaction secondary to recent, sustained use of hashish. For the three days prior to her admission the patient, who had smoked marijuana only three times in her life, had secluded herself in her bedroom at home and smoked enormous quantities of hashish, until her parents questioned her about what she was doing in her room. She confessed, and said she wished to see a psychiatrist.

On her admission to the unit, the patient presented as perplexed and somewhat depressed. She complained of feeling "confused and unreal." She stated that she had been "smoking because living at home with my parents upsets me." She had recently graduated from college in another state and had been living with her parents for the previous two weeks because, she said, "I couldn't afford to live elsewhere." She informed us that her parents had made her unhappy throughout her childhood and adolescence and that her return home following four years away at college had precipitated many painful memories. She also said that she had been in psychotherapy for four months in her senior year because, "I was running around with a lot of men and wasn't sure

I liked it. My therapist told me I was the passive victim of my own sexuality and that I was a nymphomaniac, but he seemed to expect me to give him vivid accounts of my affairs so I stopped seeing him."

Mental status examination revealed a fully oriented, intelligent young woman whose recent memory was impaired and who admitted to visual hallucinations which commenced following her use of the hallucinogens. There was no evidence of a thought disorder, but clear evidence of a preexisting borderline personality organization with pan-anxiety, poor object relations, promiscuity, multiple phobias, derealization, depersonalization, and long-standing depression.

The organic psychosis rapidly cleared after phenothiazine treatment was instituted. A treatment program was planned in which the first task was to help the patient define where she wanted to live and work. It soon became apparent that she had been searching for such structure and controls in her life. She had become convinced that school represented "total freedom and permissiveness," and that home represented "a cloistered existence involving abstinence of every kind." She arrived at the insight that she had smoked the marijuana to test her parents, "to see whether they could control me, and they have."

During a family meeting she verbalized these thoughts and feelings to her parents and told the therapist that she was "staggered" when her parents calmly stated that she could continue to live with them. Furthermore, they stated, "It is your life and we won't interfere." They hoped, however, that she would form more stable relationships with men.

It now became evident that in the manner of a classic borderline psychosis there had been ego splitting: school was seen as entirely permissive and parents were seen as entirely restricting. In addition, she was projecting her own punishing superego onto her parents, which made it impossible for her to live with them in comfort. Despite her borderline personality structure, her interest in changing and capacity for insight suggested the possibility of long-term psychodynamic psychotherapy. She was discharged to individual psychotherapy, and to begin a job that she had found while in the hospital.

A drug induced psychosis is usually easy to diagnose and the symptoms generally disappear rapidly following the institution of pharmacotherapy. Thereafter it is important to help the patient understand how the experience relates to the current life situation as well as to try to bring about some conflict resolution.

Popular mistrust of psychiatric facilities by the young can be reduced if mental health professionals demonstrate that their attitude is neither condescending nor moralistic, but that they will attempt to understand and to help. There should be no reservations about advising a patient who experienced a "bad trip" not to use drugs in the future. Arbitrary statements that drug use is wrong or illegal should be avoided: rather the advice should be that as drugs have had a deleterious effect in the past, they are likely to provoke a similar or worse reaction in the future.

Patients for Detoxification

A relatively common problem that presents to a crisis unit is the patient who is admitted for detoxification from drugs or alcohol. The defined task for the crisis unit in most cases is to withdraw the patient from the drug or from alcohol, and nothing else. Any rehabilitative program is generally undertaken by the agency that referred the patient. Should a patient be admitted who is not already in a drug or alcohol program, arrangements for such follow-up are made, where possible, on the day of admission.

DRUG WITHDRAWAL

A special problem is presented with barbiturate addiction in that it is often not suspected and is therefore overlooked. Barbiturate addicts tend to deny or minimize their addiction in much the same way that alcoholics do, and it is usually difficult to obtain an accurate history of drug use from them. Another difficulty not infrequently encountered in withdrawing an addict is that drugs may be secreted by the patient on admission or may be brought in by his or her friends.

Sudden cessation of barbiturates in a dependent individual usually results in a withdrawal syndrome that commences within 24 hours and may last for a week. The patient experiences weakness, tremulousness, restlessness, anxiety, insomnia, eyelid spasms, and elevated blood pressure at rest which reverts to a dramatic drop in blood pressure when the patient stands up suddenly. Hyperthermia, convulsions, and psychotic symptomatology may occur in untreated individuals. Barbiturate withdrawal has a significant mortality rate and it, therefore, represents a psychiatric emergency.

CASE HISTORY

Mrs. D. D., a 40-year-old, married housewife and mother of three, was admitted through the emergency room. She stated her chief complaint as, "I want to dry out." She had a history of three hospitalizations for alcoholism at a private psychiatric institution.

Her husband, an advertising executive, spent long hours away from home, and Mrs. D. filled her days with church and school activities. Their marital relationship was mediocre; she had not had intercourse with her husband for two months prior to her admission.

When she was originally evaluated in the emergency room, it was noted that there was alcohol on her breath, that her speech was slurred, and that she was tremulous. A physical examination on the unit revealed a blood pressure reading of 160/100 lying down and 110/60 standing, and she complained of dizziness on standing. Spasms of her eyelids were noted, and she admitted to insomnia the previous two nights.

At first she denied barbiturate usage, but after she was told that she could become extremely ill if she was withdrawing from barbiturates and did not receive treatment, she confessed to using approximately 800 mg of pentobarbital a day for the previous three months. Mrs. D. had apparently received monthly prescriptions for the barbiturate from her family physician, but when he left for a brief vacation, his partner refused to renew the prescription and her supply ran out.

The mental status examination revealed no evidence of a thought or perceptual disorder. A barbiturate tolerance test was performed, and she was found to be tolerant to approximately 1,000 mg of barbiturates a day. The patient was withdrawn from this level with daily decreases of 100 mg of pentobarbital. She was treated concurrently with chlordiazepoxide for withdrawal from alcohol and with thiamine for her chronic alcoholic state. The patient and her husband refused any exploration of their marital difficulties, but she was willing to accept a referral to Alcoholics Anonymous and to a drug dependency group.

THE ALCOHOLIC FOR DETOXIFICATION

Alcoholism may present as a symptom accompanying a variety of psychiatric conditions. Its treatment is complicated, difficult, and extremely frustrating to both the therapist and the patient. Because of the time limit, it is not feasible to treat all alcoholics on a crisis unit; yet the unit may provide a service for some, especially those who have social supports from family or other sources. While services a crisis unit provides such as evaluation and disposition are being performed, the patient can be detoxified.

In treating alcoholics, it is imperative to bear in mind the limitations of psychiatric treatment. These patients often have a long history of the illness and one cannot expect to undo in days what has been decades in the making. One can only try in his or her limited human way to intervene and hope that supported by the response of significant "others" in the patient's life, this may direct him to the road of longer treatment and recovery. Caution in the selection of alcoholic patients for crisis units should be used, as they may present with a myriad of medical complications, such as bleeding duodenal ulcer, alcoholic cardiomyopathy (heart disorder), aspiration pneumonia, liver failure and pancreatitis, as well as a plethora of neurological complications. No patient in delirium tremens should ever be admitted nor any other patient in whom the history or physical examination led the admitting clinician to suspect a medical complication. Most crisis units do not have the facilities, nor do most psychiatric clinicians have the necessary skills, for handling these concomitant difficulties as they arise.

CASE HISTORY

A. P., a 37-year-old, white, married, Irish Catholic father of four, was admitted to the unit from the emergency room where he had been taken by his wife following an agreement between the two that he should be hospitalized for the recurrence of a drinking problem. On admission the patient was mildly intoxicated and stated that he had been drinking for a week since his unmarried 17-year-old daughter had announced that she was pregnant and wished to get an abortion.

Mr. P. had been a member of AA for six years but had not attended meetings for the previous six months because he felt he could resist alcohol without outside help. His father and three of his uncles were alcoholics, and he had started drinking at age 16. At the time of his marriage he resolved to stop drinking but was unable to do so. He worked at the post office and was a good provider to his family but would stop off at a tavern on his way home, so that he frequently arrived home drunk and abusive. Six years prior to his current admission his wife threatened to divorce him unless he stopped drinking; he admitted himself to a state hospital for detoxification, and following discharge attended AA meetings regularly and was able to avoid the use of alcohol.

On physical examination his speech was slightly slurred, but otherwise there were no signs of neurological impairment or of chronic cardiovascular or liver disease. On mental status examination he was tearful and appeared depressed. There was no evidence of a thought or perceptual disorder. Librium 100 mg t.i.d. and a multivitamin preparation were prescribed. The day following admission the patient was completely sober and expressed remorse.

He was ashamed to face his wife and his family. But he was still reluctant to allow his daughter to have an abortion. After the staff met alone with the patient, his wife and his daughter, a couples meeting was held, and the patient and his wife decided to support their daughter's decision. It appeared that he was not so much opposed to the abortion on religious grounds as he was because he felt that his wife would think less of him for sanctioning it. When, with the help of staff, he and his wife mutually agreed that their daughter was growing up and that such a decision must include her feelings about the matter, Mr. P.'s guilt over the decision was diffused and he felt much better. He reestablished his ties with A.A. and attended a meeting while still in the hospital. The Librium was tapered by daily decreases of 50 mg, and on the seventh day of hospitalization he was discharged home.

The services provided for this patient in many respects were the same as for other patients. He was evaluated for his depression and alcoholism, the current issues in his life were clarified, communication was reestablished with his family, and a disposition was made. These tasks were relatively simple in this case since the foundations for his treatment disposition had been previously laid. With other patients, the task may be more complicated, the services of the agencies for alcoholics must not only be enlisted, but the patient must be helped to accept them.

Crisis with Potential for Violence

THE DOMESTIC CRISIS

Domestic crises frequently present to a brief treatment unit in the form of drunkenness, drug intoxication, and threats or acts of assaultive, suicidal, or homicidal behavior. Often evaluation reveals a family system in which there are chronic patterns of reinforcing maladaptive behavior by family members toward each other resulting in a tenuous equilibrium. The situation becomes acute when an internal or external force threatens to upset the system and one or more members become flagrantly symptomatic. The defined task of a crisis unit in such cases is usually clearly limited to evaluation, clarification of the immediate unsettling issues, and readjustment of the thermostat such that the equilibrium is reestablished. Once this is accomplished, it may then be possible to arrange for longer-term treatment if the family members consent to this. However, long-term intervention in the family's dynamics may cause changes which would be covertly or obviously resisted by one or more of the family members, or it may be impractical or difficult to implement such intervention ab initio as the following case illustrates.

CASE HISTORY

D. C., a 40-year-old, white, divorced, unemployed mother of six, was admitted to the crisis unit threatening, "If it goes on like this, I'm going to break my daughter's neck." Mrs. C.'s life was characterized by interminable chaos both in her family of origin and in her connubial family. She had been divorced from her third husband for two years and alternated between a state of being able to cope with the rearing of her children, in which, according to all sources, "she was like a lamb," and short-lived tirades against all and sundry, particularly when under the influence of alcohol. Her youngest brother, who lived in a nearby town, would occasionally visit her on the weekends, at which times he would bring her a bottle of vodka. D. C. was constantly in a battle with one or other of her children. This time it appeared to be her 14-year-old daughter, who she stated, "shoots off her mouth at me and won't do the dishes." There was no history of a previous psychiatric hospitalization or consultation, and there was no evidence of a major psychiatric disorder other than her explosive behavior when under the influence of alcohol. She admitted to getting drunk five or six times a year, but denied regular use of alcohol.

It was decided that the patient should be interviewed alone and with her 14-year-old daughter and that her social network should be carefully assessed. During interviews with her it emerged that her problems with her daughter had commenced six months previously when the daughter, who was very attractive, began to date and "seemed to be having a good time" while D. C. "sat home and slaved with the dishes." When the daughter was interviewed, she was a somewhat hostile and defiant adolescent girl who stated, "If my mother thinks she can stop me dating, she has another guess coming." She confirmed that her mother only drank when her brother brought her vodka, which was not more than five or six times a year. A subsequent meeting with both mother and daughter revealed that neither was going to give way, and neither made any moves toward attempting to understand what was going on with the other, or between them. It became clear that psychotherapy would not help, so attention was turned to the question of how the patient coped with her role as mother and father for six children. A community worker was involved in the case, and together with the patient made two home visits. This revealed the fact that there had been no heat in the home for the past month because of an unpaid bill and that the family had been boiling water on the stove in order to bathe. With the help of the community worker, the patient was able to get the bill paid and have a homemaker help her with the chores.

A neighbor volunteered to stay with the young children one evening a week so that the patient could attend A. A. meetings. The patient's brother was contacted by phone, and he agreed not to bring his sister alcohol in the future. On the day of her discharge, the patient told us that she felt much better and that she now realized that she had been "dumping" on her daughter, that the boy her daughter was dating was "a gentleman," and that she would not let things "slide" again.

The staff was aware of the very real possibility that one or more members of this family might become symptomatic at some point in the future and that this, indeed, often does occur despite the employment of traditional long-term family or individual psychotherapy. Therefore, a time-limited intervention into the family system was the treatment modality of choice.

The concept of *episodic treatment* alluded to in the treatment of chronic schizophrenics also applies to the treatment of families which maintain a pathological and generally unsatisfying equilibrium. Such families, it may be assumed, will have periodical flare-ups often contemporaneously with the anticipation of a fantasized or real change in the family system, such as one member leaving home to marry. At such times it is hoped that given a past history of successful intervention at times of crisis, a family will return to the mental health center for the help it may require.

THE HOMICIDAL PATIENT

The admission of a homicidal patient to a crisis unit is usually anxiety-provoking to the staff at all levels. After the admission of a homicidal patient has been announced, there is often a barrage of questions and a flurry of activities aimed at controlling some of the anxiety.

Usually, when homicidal ideation develops, it is in the context of specific interpersonal relationships and is not diffuse. In the evaluation of homicidal patients it is often possible to define the specific cause of the homicidal ideas. A remedy can often be worked out, either through intrapsychic change or more frequently through environmental manipulation. In performing the evaluation, it is essential to determine the factors that weaken the patient's controls, e.g., drugs or alcohol. The therapeutic thrust can then be directed toward helping the patient and his family implement ways in which those factors might be avoided or minimized.

The patient who is diffusely homicidal is not appropriate for a crisis unit and is best managed at a facility which has the necessary structure built in to control homicidal behavior, e.g., a maximum security ward at a state hospital.

Organic pathology, such as temporal lobe dysfunction, should always be considered, and it is good practice to obtain a routine electroencephalogram in all cases involving homicidal ideation. Once the patient's symptoms are understood in the context of the history, management can be quite straightforward, as the following case demonstrates.

CASE HISTORY

H. P., a 20-year-old, white, single male was referred to the unit by a local psychiatrist who had treated him for the previous six months on a once-a-week basis in individual psychotherapy. The patient had sought treatment because of vague anxiety, loneliness, and difficulty in deciding on his long-term career plans. He was in the Air Force Reserves and spent one weekend each month with them and two weeks every year on active duty at a training camp.

A month before he was due to report to camp, he told his psychiatrist that he hated the service and could not tolerate the regimentation and discipline. He subsequently stated that he had made up his mind to shoot the commanding officer and anyone else who might attempt to keep him at the post. This developed into a fixed idea, which so convinced the psychiatrist that he referred the patient to the crisis unit a week before he was due to leave for the camp.

The patient had been the child of a planned and wanted pregnancy and was delivered without mishap. His milestones were achieved at the normal age, and he had average grades at school. His father was somewhat of a strict disciplinarian and always made him feel inept. He described his mother as kind and affectionate.

Masturbation commenced at age 12 and was accompanied by heterosexual fantasies. At age 13 and 14 he engaged in mutual masturbation with male acquaintances; there was, however, no history of homosexual activity beyond this. He seldom dated and had never gone beyond necking and petting. Following graduation from high school, he found employment at a local factory and attended night courses in psychology at a state college.

Throughout his history ran a theme of poor relationships with authority figures; he was never able to assert himself. An example of this was his response to what he felt to be an unjustifiable punishment meted out to him by a teacher. He had brooded for a month, could not concentrate, slept poorly, and became preoccupied with the thought of poisoning the teacher. These thoughts became quite intense, and he was relieved when the teacher was promoted to vice-principal and a substitute took over the class.

The patient denied drug or alcohol use and seemed to have good impulse control. The mental status examination was remarkable in terms of flattened affect, circumstantial thinking and an encapsulated delusional system in which the Air Force—and the commander in particular—were seen as tormentors who were intent on harming or killing him. He felt that the only way out would be to shoot the commander, and the intensity of his murderous thoughts towards this person was quite alarming.

An electroencephalogram was obtained and was reported normal. On the basis of the history and of the mental status examination, a diagnosis of paranoid schizophrenia was made. Phenothiazines brought about some reduction in the intensity of the homicidal thoughts but did not remove them. Two days after admission, the unit commander was contacted and was informed about the situation. He readily provided information as to how the patient's discharge from the Air Force might be secured, and this was effected within a few days. The patient was then discharged home, to be maintained on the phenothiazine by his psychiatrist.

THE SUICIDAL PATIENT

The evaluation of a patient's suicidal potential plays an important role in the determination of whether a patient can be treated as an outpatient or needs to be hospitalized. Admission to a crisis unit is often occasioned by actual suicide attempts or concern by clinicians about imminent ones. Obviously, not everyone who talks of suicide or even gestures seriously intends to kill himself. While the ability to unequivocally state that a patient would not take his life is not always possible, there are certain epidemiological, psychological, and sociological factors which facilitate such evaluations. (See "Evaluation of Suicidal and Homicidal Potential, page 60).

CASE HISTORY

S. P., a 65-year-old, white, divorced, agnostic, childless, retired school teacher, was transferred to the crisis unit from a medical ward where she was being treated for an overdose of a tricyclic antidepressant.

The patient was born the third of a family of six children in a small midwestern town. Both parents lived to be quite old, and there was no history of psychiatric illness in the family, although her mother had been mildly depressed after two of her pregnancies. The patient was brought up on her parents' farm in adequate socioeconomic circumstances. While her siblings were interested in remaining in the area and married local townsmen, she went off to a small state teachers college. At college, she met her husband, five years her senior, who was of a similar background. They moved east to work, but after ten years of marriage were divorced because she did not want children, and he began an affair with another woman. Although she dated intermittently after the divorce, she never remarried and only once had a relationship that included sexual intercourse.

She was active in several local political and social organizations that met at the school in which she taught, and all of her friends were in some way related to these groups. Following her retirement, six months prior to admission, she gradually stopped attending the groups and became increasingly worried about finances and about her worth as an individual. Four months prior to admission she began to lose her appetite, and had lost twenty pounds at the time of admission. In addition, she began to have difficulty falling asleep and awoke each morning around four o'clock. One week prior to admission she went to her internist who prescribed a tricyclic antidepressant. Two days prior to admission she took the overdose and was found by a neighbor who stopped by because she had become concerned when the patient said earlier in the day that she did not expect to see her anymore. After two days of medical treatment in a general hospital, she was transferred to the crisis unit.

On admission to the ward the patient appeared tearful, depressed, and remorseful over her "evil" act. She claimed that she did not want to die but did not see how she could "continue to be a parasite." After several meetings, it became clear that the patient had centered nearly her entire life around her teaching career, and having retired she felt that she could no longer be a useful member of the community.

Much to the staff's pleasant surprise, several of the patient's old friends began to appear on the ward, having been informed by the patient's neighbor of her illness. They expressed surprise at the patient's fears, and were happy to have her continue her work in the political and social groups. In addition, the crisis staff helped direct her to a hospital where she was able to get a volunteer position.

After two weeks of rallying the patient's social supports coupled with the reinitiation of the patient's tricyclic medication, she appeared more optimistic, denied any further suicidal ideation, and was able to be discharged to an outpatient medication and support group.

THE MELODRAMA

Not infrequently patients are admitted to a crisis unit following the exhibition of dramatic suicidal threats or gestures that cause others to be concerned about their safety. These patients, often young women, employ self-destructive behavior primarily for its communicative value within the context of their interpersonal relationships. Rarely do they actually intend to kill themselves. The threat or actual attempt to harm themselves is employed manipulatively in an attempt to achieve a goal such as preventing a lover from ending a relationship. The defined task of a crisis unit in such cases is to assess the true suicidal potential of such a patient and to assist him or her in the development of more mature and direct ways of communicating.

CASE HISTORY

M. P., an 18-year-old, white, single freshman at a small, denominational, Eastern woman's college, was admitted to the crisis unit from the emergency room, where she had been brought by a roommate following the ingestion of twenty aspirin tablets and half a pint of wine. There was no history of previous psychiatric treatment.

The patient had begun dating a 21-year-old senior at another local college six months prior to admission. After one month of "necking and heavy petting," they began having intercourse once to twice a week, but she was unable to achieve climax. She had had no previous sexual experience but had begun on the contraceptive pill on entering college and so was not pregnant. Her boyfriend, about to graduate, had planned to attend a professional school several hundred miles from the patient, and as his graduation was drawing near, the relationship had been winding down, at his initiative. On the night of admission he had told her that he did not wish to see her again. Following this, she left her dormitory and, in the presence of her roommate, took the overdose of aspirin and wine.

Past personal history, medical history, and mental status examination were unremarkable. Following admission and initial interviewing, the patient was observed on the unit and found to be somewhat hystrionic in her manner and superficial in her interpersonal relations. But no major psychopathology could be detected. She stated that she had had no intention of harming herself seriously. The gesture had been impulsive, related directly to her feelings after the boyfriend's announcement. While protesting that she did not wish for the staff to contact him because it would make him feel guilty to discover that she was in the hospital, he learned of the hospitalization and appeared on the unit within 24 hours of admission to see her. At that time he met with a staff member and explained that he did wish to terminate the relationship but that her behavior made him feel very guilty. He was told that he should attempt to decide what he wished to do and that he should communicate his plans to the patient while she was on the unit. He met with her, said that he did not want to continue the relationship, and then left the unit. Thirty-six hours later the patient felt considerably better and asked to be discharged to return to school.

M. P. was discharged and returned for three follow-up appointments. By the end of that time she had found a new boyfriend and declined further treatment. She saw her overdose as an angry and desperate attempt to hold onto her boyfriend by making him feel guilty for wanting to leave her.

Although this case is typical of some admissions to crisis wards, many such cases are seen in emergency rooms. The decision to hospitalize such a patient depends on a number of factors including the availability for assessment of the protagonists in the drama, the experience of the evaluating individual, and the possibility of obtaining a good history and mental status examination at the time of the initial contact. The latter is often difficult and can be impossible if the patient is heavily intoxicated.

Once admitted, it is imperative that a complete history be secured to rule out major psychopathology. The family history of such patients often indicates that the patient has had exposure to individuals who have behaved in comparable ways in similar situations. Usually, the message intended to be conveyed by the gesture is easily ascertained once a full history is obtained, and it should be made explicit to the patient and discussed.

It is generally undesirable to attempt to assist in the implicit goal of maintaining a relationship against the wishes of another party. Such attempts rarely succeed and if they do the contract for continuing the relationship is based on dishonesty, manipulation, and guilt. Not only will this provide an unhealthy climate for the couple to continue their relationship, but it will reinforce the patient's belief that suicidal behavior in the future will bring equal rewards. Moreover, such patients tend to be fickle, sexually provocative, and somewhat shallow in their relationships, and no sooner has one stormy relationship ended than a new one is embarked on.

THE LEGAL REFERRAL

Sometimes patients involved with some part of the legal system are referred to a crisis unit. The task requested by a lawyer, a judge, or whoever is involved, is to observe and evaluate the person's behavior. While most forensic psychiatric evaluations can be performed on an outpatient basis, the longitudinal 24-hour observation by clinicians skilled in observing nuances of behavior is obviously advantageous. Such evaluations are not only valuable to the courts but help to insure that the patient's ultimate disposition is suitable to his condition. While some diagnostic enigmas may present, most are relatively straightforward.

CASE HISTORY

L. R., a 15-year-old, white, single, Protestant ninth-grade student, was referred to the crisis unit by a private psychiatrist who was asked to evaluate the patient by his lawyer. Two days prior to admission the patient had attempted to kill his nine-year-old sister.

The patient was the second of three children, having a sister two years older, in addition to the one mentioned. His parents stated that he was never very active as a child, always sought to be alone, and shunned contact sports. Although he did average school work, he was considered "queer" and "odd" by his classmates because of grotesque stories he would tell for their attention. He liked to bury dead animals and went through elaborate funeral rituals when doing so. His only extracurricular activity was a science club. He never dated and had no close friends. He denied any history of drug use. He had masturbated about once a week for two years prior to admission, but this had increased in frequency to two to three times a week in the month preceding admission.

Two nights prior to admission he was babysitting with his younger sister while his parents attended a dance at their country club. After the two had eaten a meal and their parents had left, his sister retired to her bedroom and the patient to his. He spent some time alone in his room while his "mind went blank." Then suddenly without forethought, he grabbed a bicycle chain and ran into his sister's room and tried to strangle her. After this failed, he took a knife he had purchased earlier in the week and stabbed her several times, causing the collapse of one lung and lacerations to the face and thigh. He then ran out of the house into a wood surrounding it and remained there until he was apprehended the next day by the police and taken to jail. There he signed a confession admitting to the assault.

On admission the patient appeared withdrawn and guarded. He exhibited blocking and his affect was most inappropriate. He smiled as he recounted the story of the assault on his sister. A complete neurological examination was performed in addition to obtaining several ancillary diagnostic tests such as an electroencephalogram, lumbar puncture, and brain scan. Further historical data gathered on the unit from the patient, his parents, and older sister coupled with the observations of his behavior on the ward confirmed the diagnosis of schizophrenia. A mildly abnormal electroencephalogram was suggestive of the possibility of an organic component. The rest of the diagnostic tests and neurological examination, however, were grossly within normal limits. Over a period of ten days the patient remained vague and guarded. We were unable to ascertain what had prompted the assault. He was therefore transferred to a long-term psychiatric facility for further evaluation and treatment. A complete summary of his evaluation was sent to his lawyer, with the permission of his family.

An important part of this patient's treatment on the crisis unit was the work with his parents and older sister. (His younger sister was hospitalized on a surgical ward following the assault and eventually recovered from her wounds.) The focus of the family meetings, after the necessary historical information was obtained and the transfer to another hospital effected, was in helping them deal with their feelings surrounding the incident. Not only had their young daughter narrowly escaped a violent death, but her assailant was their own son. The opportunity given to them to ventilate their feelings, and the staff's help in the immediate planning of their future, is an example of the preventive psychiatric function crisis wards can serve. While the unit's involvement with the family terminated upon the transfer of the patient, it was suggested to the referral hospital that continued family work, which should include the patient's younger sister after her discharge, would be necessary if the family was to be successfully reintegrated after the crisis had resolved.

External Stress Crisis

THE ACUTE GRIEF REACTION

One of the earliest applications of the crisis mode of therapeutic intervention was that described for the treatment of grief reactions following loss. (See first chapter, "The History of Crisis Intervention.") When mourning reaches pathological proportions because of either its intensity or duration, referral to a crisis unit may result.

CASE HISTORY

G. R. is a 28-year-old, white, married mother of two who presented six weeks after her two-year-old daughter died following surgery for a congenital heart defect. The patient was referred to the crisis unit by the family pediatrician, who had been contacted by the patient's husband.

Mrs. R. had no previous psychiatric history and had been in good physical health all of her life. She had had normal pregnancies and deliveries of her children. The youngest, now deceased, had difficulty from birth requiring special care, and failed to thrive. The parents had known since the first month that her prognosis was guarded but at considerable cost had sought the most expert treatment for her. They had been advised to have the surgery although it was deemed risky. The alternative, unfortunately, was almost certain decline over the next several months. With difficulty, they decided upon a date for the surgery. Two days following the procedure the child died suddenly from heart failure.

Following this the patient became depressed, with frequent cry-ing jags. She had great difficulty sleeping and was unable to keep from crying while caring for her two other children. Her husband was supportive and concerned, and when the reaction persisted beyond the second week, he arranged for his mother to stay with the family. The relief from the routine work pressure around the house did not help the patient's symptoms, and in desperation Mr. R. finally sought the counsel of their pediatrician. At first, the doctor attempted to sedate Mrs. R., but when this proved ineffective and she began describing herself as a "burden," he referred her to the crisis unit.

Upon admission, the patient was depressed, but not suicidal, and very eager to talk. When encouraged, she ventilated the feelings of guilt she felt for having had a sick baby in the first place, for allowing the opera-tion, for not caring adequately for her family prior to and since the death of the daughter, and for not being able to pull herself out of the doldrums. She queried whether, in fact, she had unconsciously wanted her daughter to die. She questioned what people thought of her, espe-cially her children, her mother-in-law, and her husband. If permitted, she would talk on about these themes for an hour or more, at the end of which time she would temporarily appear better.

The patient remained in the hospital for eight days. At the end of this time her sleep had improved considerably and her crying was confined to two or three brief periods per day when something would remind her of her daughter. She took several visiting passes home and was amazed to find that her mother-in-law was understanding rather than vindictive. She was gratified to find her husband was pleased to see her and relieved at her improvement. She had found it easy to believe that the crisis staff would be accepting of her grieving but prior to her passes she doubted her family's ability to do so.

After discharge the patient returned to see her primary clinician on the unit once a week for a month. Then she told the clinician that she no longer felt a need for further help and would talk to her minister if any problem came up in the future. The clinician responded by sup-porting her decision and stated that a therapist at the mental health center would be available for consultation should future problems arise.

The vast majority of grief reactions do not require psychiatric hospi-talization. Most individuals contend with a loss by utilizing the support of family, friends, or clergy who are generally quite successful in getting them through the critical period of grieving.

THE TRANSIENT SITUATIONAL CRISIS

The patient experiencing a transient situational crisis presents with anxiety or hopelessness and a sense of inability to cope with a particular situation. Often, the presenting complaint is that of insomnia, and frequently a somatic symptom such as dyspepsia, diarrhea, or headache will be in evidence. Sometimes the patient in a situational crisis will actually complain of feeling confused or "mixed up" and will request a few days on the crisis unit to "pull myself together."

Most often these cases can be successfully treated on an outpatient basis, provided that the patient's symptoms are not crippling and adequate supports are available in the form of concerned family or friends. Occasionally, however, the severity of the symptoms or the lack of resources makes a brief hospitalization mandatory, as the following case illustrates.

CASE HISTORY

T. D., a 73-year-old, single, retired, Jewish male, was admitted to the crisis unit through the efforts of a social worker attached to a family agency in New Haven. Mr. D.'s chief complaint at the time of admission was, "I don't have anywhere to live and I haven't been sleeping too well."

Approximately a month prior to his admission, Mr. D. had been informed by his landlady that she intended to raise his rent by $10 per week because she felt she had been undercharging him for years. At about the same time he had learned that a part-time job as an elevator operator, which brought a small supplementary addition to his Social Security check, would no longer be available because the company was installing automatic elevators. He suddenly took to his bed and refused to eat—"a hunger strike," as he later described it. His landlady contacted a family agency, and a social worker was sent to visit him. She found that she "had nowhere to put the poor man" and decided to contact the crisis unit "on the offchance that you'd take him."

On admission Mr. D. presented as a somewhat crusty, but likeable, elderly man. A comprehensive psychiatric history and mental status examination gave no evidence of major psychopathology. A social work student expressed interest in the case and became his primary clinician. Her initial task was to overcome some of the resistance that Mr. D.

expressed about moving from his old apartment. After a trusting relationship had been established with the clinician, the patient was encouraged to disclose his financial resources in detail. A considerable nest egg was revealed and this provided the wherewithal for him to be accepted at a modern, well-run home for the elderly. Following one month of supportive outpatient follow-up, Mr. D. was in good physical and mental health, and his treatment was terminated.

This patient clearly required assistance in dealing with specific external environmental stresses, namely his living and job situations. It is important to remember, particularly in the context of crisis intervention, that hospitalization is not synonymous with mental illness. People are referred to psychiatric hospitals for a variety of reasons including scarce resources, abandonment, physical illness, and family fatigue. Attention must therefore be paid to the precipitants of the referral rather than assuming that mere admission is evidence of pathology.

THE THERAPY CRISIS

The development of a strong interpersonal bond between a patient and his therapist is an important part of many of the so-called psychological therapies. This aspect of psychotherapy is unfortunately a double-edged sword. While it is often a powerful tool in effecting personality change, feelings arising out of the relationship can lead to difficulty, even with the most scrupulous and experienced of therapists. There are times when the vicissitudes of therapy threaten to overwhelm the patient, and the therapist may then have to consider hospitalizing the patient for a brief period. This kind of situation classically arises around a major disruption in therapy, such as a therapist's vacation or the impending or actual termination of therapy. The forces at work may, however, be more subtle, such as when a patient "acts out" around what he perceives as hostile or overly seductive behavior on the part of the therapist. A brief hospitalization can afford both patient and therapist the opportunity to assess and clarify the issues, or it can be used to effect a transfer to another therapist or another therapy modality, such as a group.

CASE HISTORY

Miss T. C., a 23-year-old, single elementary school teacher was admitted from the emergency room with a chief complaint of, "I've been feeling anxious and have been thinking that life isn't worth living." She had been brought to the emergency room by her roommate, who became alarmed when the patient told her that she felt lonely and depressed and wanted to hurt herself in some way. Miss C. presented as a bright, attractive but somewhat disconsolate girl who stated that she could not understand why she was feeling upset. During the course of a comprehensive psychiatric history, she revealed that she had been seeing a psychotherapist for the previous six months because of her inability to handle relationships with men.

One week prior to her hospitalization, her therapist had left for a 10-day vacation. He had informed her about the vacation a month before, and when she pressed him for details, he said that he was taking his wife and family to an island in the Caribbean. During the following session the patient requested an increase in therapy to twice a week. She did not understand the basis for her request except that, "I wanted to see more of him!" The therapist took the request up on a manifest level and told her that he did not have the additional time available.

The patient's past history was unremarkable except for the fact that she had been involved in three intense heterosexual relationships which all ended because, she said, "They all became too dependent on me and I couldn't stand that." After she ended the last relationship, she decided to consult a psychotherapist: "I wanted to understand more about myself and how I relate to men." She described her therapist as "strong, mature, and very attractive," and she discovered after a few sessions that she had become very attached to him. She began to think how much she would like to be married to someone like him and, although she was much sought after, she stopped dating. When she learned about his vacation, she felt hurt and unhappy, and after he refused her request for the additional hour she became, as she put it, "angry and resentful, and started thinking about hurting myself." Miss C. now felt that no one could help her and that her therapist would in all likelihood not want to continue treating her because she had been hospitalized in his absence.

On the third day of hospitalization the therapist returned from his vacation. The patient was initially adamant that he not be contacted while she was on the unit, but her protestations were overcome. With the announcement of the therapist's impending arrival on the unit, there came a flurry of activity in front of her mirror. After she had met with the therapist, she felt that "our problems have been worked out" and felt ready to return to him as an outpatient.

The therapist met with the staff during rounds and agreed that the hospitalization was directly related to issues in therapy. He acknowledged that the patient's admission was probably aimed at punishing and testing him and felt that he may have indeed "fueled the transference" by not directing the patient to strengthen her relationships outside therapy. In addition, he felt that he had turned down the patient's request for a second hour in a somewhat arbitrary fashion instead of interpreting it in terms of her response to the announcement of his upcoming vacation.

It was suggested to the therapist that Miss C.'s dependency needs might be diluted if she were to begin group therapy concurrent with her individual therapy. It was left to the therapist to discuss this plan and its rationale with the patient, and she readily agreed to it.

Life Cycle Crisis

THE ADOLESCENT IN CRISIS

Adolescents are referred to the crisis unit for reasons ranging from drug abuse, antisocial behavior, sexual behavior with social or legal ramifications, and mood disturbances to schizophrenic symptomatology. Resolution of the difficulties confronting an adolescent and his family is usually not possible during a brief hospitalization. Rather, the tasks that can be accomplished are, as with other patients, evaluation, symptom reduction, and referral for further treatment. With adolescents, the evaluation should include the whole family, as the following case demonstrates.

CASE HISTORY

A. C. is a 17-year-old, black, unmarried mother of a one-year-old son. She was admitted to the crisis unit from the emergency room, to which she had been brought by her two sisters following the ingestion of six sleeping pills. Her chief complaint at the time of admission was, "My mother won't take care of my baby for me, and I want to go back to school. I wish I was dead."

Three weeks prior to admission the patient, who was living with her mother, her child, and her sisters in her mother's apartment, told her mother that she wished to return to school to complete her education. Her mother responded by telling her to stay home and look after her child—"like you're supposed to." This constituted a reversal of a promise that her mother had made during her pregnancy, when she had said that A. could return to school when the baby was a year old. A heated argument ensued, during which A.'s mother threatened her with a carving knife. Hours later A. told her sisters that she had taken an overdose of medication, and they brought her to the emergency room.

A comprehensive psychiatric history was unremarkable save for the fact that A. had conceived the child out of wedlock shortly before her sixteenth birthday and had herself chosen not to get married because, she said, "I didn't like the boy's family." Mental status examination revealed no evidence of schizophrenia or significant depression. The initial treatment plan was for meetings with the patient and her mother separately, to be followed by meetings with them together. During the interviews with A. she expressed a strong interest in returning to school. Her academic record was excellent, and she hoped to become a teacher.

A.'s mother stated that she felt she was too old to have to look after a small child. She revealed that one of her other daughters was pregnant as well and said, "I don't want them all to believe that they can take advantage of me like that." It became clear that Mrs. C., who previously had viewed A. as her favorite, in fact strongly identified with A. She had unresolved feelings about A.'s pregnancy because she herself had had an abortion at age 16. When A. became pregnant, Mrs. C. refused to allow her to have an abortion.

Although Mrs. C. behaved very appropriately toward the staff, she was not able to tolerate a conjoint meeting with her daughter without outbursts of anger and threats of violence towards her. The staff worked intensively with mother and daughter in an effort to overcome the impasse but after a few days it became obvious that this was a fruitless endeavor. To make matters worse, A. threatened to go to school come what may, stating, "If I leave my son at home my mother will just have to look after him." Mrs. C.'s response was that if that happened, she would call the Protective Services in an effort to have the child placed in a foster home.

At this point a psychiatric aide suggested that the local Welfare Moms be contacted since it is the endeavor of this organization to prevent an offspring of a family receiving welfare from being taken from the family. Representatives of the Welfare Moms were invited onto the unit. After telling both mother and daughter that "we aren't going to put up with your nonsense," they told them directly that one of them would visit the home every day to help out with the care of the baby and would make sure that the patient took at least partial responsibility for the baby's care. At a final interview, Mrs. C. recanted and told her daughter that she would allow her to return to school. A. was then discharged to her home to make arrangements for this.

Most noteworthy when adolescents are admitted to a crisis unit is that the evaluation must include information about the family and contact with the family must be made. In A.'s case, the mother not only figured in precipitating the crisis, but her own conflicts were obstacles to its resolution. Only after the full evaluation can a prediction be made about the kind of treatment and referral. Some families are amenable to family therapy alone or combined with individual treatment for the adolescent. This was not the case with this family.

Finally, when definite treatment of a family situation is not a possibility, it is not necessarily predictive of chronic difficulties. Family patterns do change as members marry or leave for other reasons. While the family constellation represented in this case is not a stable one, it does not follow that the patient will never be able to achieve a stable life for herself when she finishes school and, as is likely, leaves home. Thus, all that is maladaptive does not have to be treated. The lack of stability can sometimes be an impetus for change irrespective of therapy.

THE ABORTION EVALUATION

The need for a therapeutic abortion often comes at a time when the patient—perhaps an adolescent—and her family are in turmoil. Conflicting feelings of such an intense nature may be aroused in her, her parents, siblings, and sometimes close relatives that the psychiatrist who is called in for a consultation on an outpatient basis may be confronted with an overwhelming task. The evaluation should establish who is actually making the request (e.g., parent, child) and from whom the pressure for an abortion is coming (e.g., parent, boyfriend); and in the light of this information, what the response of the patient and her family is likely to be to a decision to permit or refuse the abortion.

It is important to keep in mind that there is little evidence demonstrating long-term detrimental effects on women undergoing abortions (Aarons, 1967; Meyerowitz *et al.*, 1971; Simon and Senturia, 1966, 1967; Sloane, 1969; Whittington, 1970).

From the standpoint of the staff, nursing personnel sometimes experience difficulties of a personal nature in working with such patients, and it is not unusual for the patient to become the target of intense hostility (Char and McDermott, 1972). It is, therefore, mandatory on a crisis unit to encourage those most intimately connected with the patient to have the opportunity to ventilate their feelings about the abortion to an experienced clinician, his or her task being to ensure that the patient is treated with sympathy and respect.

CASE HISTORY

A. E., a 16-year-old, white, Protestant, sophomore in high school, was admitted to the unit by a psychiatrist who had been consulted by a gynecologist to assess the patient for an abortion. He had found that the patient and her family were unable to reach an agreement and thought that the issues might better be clarified in an inpatient setting.

The patient was an attractive, intelligent girl who was found on examination to be ten to eleven weeks pregnant. She stated that she thought that she wanted an abortion but just couldn't make up her mind about it. Her history revealed her to be resourceful, a friendly girl who did well at school and had many friends. Her milestones were achieved at the normal time, and her early development appeared to be entirely within normal limits. Six months prior to admission, she started to date a young classmate whom she claimed she did not love. She had intercourse with him on three occasions to "find out what it was like" and then stopped because "I realized I was cheapening myself and I had a hunch I might be pregnant."

Mental status examination was deemed within normal limits. A treatment plan was devised whereby the patient would meet with her primary clinician daily, and another clinician would meet with her parents to evaluate their feelings and conflicts about their daughter.

During the course of her interviews, A. was able to identify her main conflict as being her relationship with her mother, who she said, "started telling me when I was a kid that all that boys want from girls is sex, that she would never trust me with boys, and that I would probably get pregnant by the time I was sixteen." She stated that after she developed the steady relationship with the boy who impregnated her, her mother would ask her after each date, "How far did you go?" "I made up my mind that if that was going to be her attitude, I might as well get pregnant."

When the parents were interviewed, it became evident that Mrs. E. had indeed acted in a controlling, hostile, and deprecating way toward her daughter, probably as the result of having been herself forced into marriage because of an unwanted pregnancy when she was eighteen. A.'s pregnancy had evoked painful memories in her parents: Mr. E. stated, "In some way we're going through the same kinds of things again as when we decided to get married."

During a conjoint meeting with both A. and her parents it became clear that after a period of heated arguments at home A. had made up her mind that she wanted an abortion, but that her parents' ambivalence had impeded them all from taking action. At a family meeting, Mrs. E. said that her husband could never make up his mind about anything and that she was tired of bearing the responsibility for every decision. She told her husband, "I decided that this time you'd have to experience some guilt along with me." At eighteen she too had wanted an abortion but her husband had procrastinated until it was too late. Mr. E. expressed his wish that A. finish school and go to college. He said that she was too young to look after a child and that, indeed, she should have the abortion.

At this point it appeared that A. was still conflicted and when interviewed alone said that the gynecologist she had consulted had been brusque, judgmental, and moralistic. The clinician suggested that the family might agree for her to see another gynecologist. She seemed relieved, and said, "It was such a hassle to get them to take me to see him in the first place that I thought they'd never let me see another."

A female staff member was then assigned the task of explaining the exact nature of the procedure to the patient and allaying some of her anxieties concerning the possible aftereffects, such as her fear that she would be left infertile. This clinician visited A. on the gynecology ward after the abortion and undertook to follow the family for a course of brief treatment after A.'s discharge from the hospital.

This case demonstrates many principles common to crisis therapy. Not infrequently one member of the family may be formally identified as a patient by other family members who themselves are seeking help. The number of available staff and the crisis unit's orientation toward evaluating the family system allows issues and conflicts to surface which may go unnoticed in a strictly individual approach. The use of separate evaluation of parents and adolescent creates the necessary therapeutic bonds of trust that may not develop if the same clinician sees both. With the minimization of the fear that a "guilty" party may be identified, communication is facilitated which can serve as the basis for initiation of family therapy. Family members who were hostile to any outside intervention into the difficulties confronting them in their own homes may acclimate to the presence of a neutral figure who can help clarify the issues.

Finally, there are problems which may touch on unresolved conflicts or awaken those ostensibly solved in staff members. Problems such as abortion, adultery, and violence often arouse anxiety in staff members which may be defended against in a variety of ways, some of which may be detrimental to good patient care. Members of the staff evincing signs of conflict should be identified by more senior staff members. If they themselves are unaware of their difficulty, other staff members should in a sensitive way minimize these staff members involvements. It is always important that a clinician's personal conflicts and needs not interfere with the quality of psychiatric treatment afforded by a treatment facility. While a clear sense of one's own value system is a mark of a mature individual, one's values and mores must not interfere with the equitable and sensitive rendering of mental health services to all who may request it.

THE POSTPARTUM PSYCHOSIS

Psychoses in the puerperium have been estimated to be as high as 1 in every 400 to 1,000 childbirths (Harris, 1950). Although both parents will respond in a variety of ways to the advent of a new child, the combination of the endocrinological and psychological changes concomitant with the pregnancy and delivery may prove especially stressful for the new mother. Both schizophreniform and affective disorders may occur in addition to a spectrum of less disabling psychological changes ranging from a mild depression to transient anxiety states.

Possible etiological factors that have been suggested as playing a role include toxic and metabolic changes, exacerbation of latent psychoses, and psychodynamic factors such as ambivalence about taking care of the child or resumption of sexual relationships following a period of abstinence. While puerperal reactions may continue for several months, requiring longer hospitalization, they often clear in a few days without any significant impairment of functioning, as the following case illustrates.

CASE HISTORY

P. P., a 25-year-old, white, married, Catholic schoolteacher was admitted in a state of agitation and excitement one week after the birth of her first son. Her family doctor felt unable to handle her on an outpatient basis so she was referred to the crisis unit.

The patient was one of two children born to parents who were in their late twenties at the time of her birth, and who were still living together. Her father was a foreman in a factory and her mother a housewife. She was raised in comfortable but not affluent socioeconomic circumstances. The parents denied any history of interpersonal difficulty while the patient was growing up, but the patient reported that she and her mother fought persistently over her dating in high school and early college. She did well in high school and then went on to a local state college while continuing to live at home.

She graduated at 21 and began work as a schoolteacher, which she continued until her pregnancy. Two years prior to admission she met the man who was to become her husband. He was a year older than her and worked as an engineer. After ten months of dating, they became engaged. Her parents opposed any plans of marriage, however, because her husband was to go into active duty in the army in three months. Despite the objections, they married and during a leave shortly before he was to transfer overseas, she conceived. After her husband left she decided to live alone. Two weeks before the delivery her husband called, and she told him that although she was saddened he could not be present, she was "overjoyed" at the prospect of the birth.

The few days following the birth were unremarkable, but on the fourth day she became increasingly excited and burst into fits of laughter. When her grandmother came to visit, the patient told her in confidence that she was the Virgin Mary and that her conception had been immaculate. Her family doctor began her on a phenothiazine, but she was unable to sleep despite what seemed to him to be an adequate dose, so he referred her to the crisis unit.

On admission the patient appeared delusional and excited, and her affect was inappropriate. Although she denied that she had said she was the Virgin Mary, she stated that there was "something very special" happening to her and that only when God felt it was appropriate to reveal the secret she would.

The diagnostic impression was that of a schizophreniform postpartum psychosis and the medication that her family doctor had begun was raised to doses adequate to control the symptomatology. Although he had, indeed, begun her on the appropriate medication, the dose had been much less than that generally used with such patients; when the dose was raised, she rapidly recompensated and began sleeping eight hours a night.

Shortly after admission her husband was contacted via the Red Cross, and he was flown home within a few days. While he was in transit and the patient was recovering, her parents were seen and plans were made to help in the care of her child. Although she hoped eventually to be able to handle him alone, she acknowledged an ambivalent desire to do so, especially in the absence of her husband. When her husband returned, plans were made for him to complete his service near the town where his wife was living so he could spend evenings with her. They discussed a plan whereby her parents and he would work together with the patient in the care of the child. After a week and a half, the patient's baby was brought onto the ward so that the mother–child interaction could be observed. After the staff felt satisfied that the patient would be able to care for her child, given the support of her husband and parents, she was discharged to be followed on medication by her family physician.

THE GERIATRIC PATIENT

Geriatric patients represent a subgroup which is probably more frequently encountered on crisis units than on more traditional medium-length treatment facilities. This can be attributed to the fact that a short-term unit can be more easily used for evaluation and disposition —the two tasks most frequently asked of a unit in reference to such patients. It is important for clinicians on such units to realize that the norms for behavior which may be applied to other age groups are not necessarily appropriate for elderly patients. For instance, a certain amount of paranoia and memory disturbance (especially for recent events) is a frequent accompaniment of the aging process. In addition, it is unusual to see a neurosis de novo in an older person with a stable premorbid adjustment.

It is often overlooked that even a "grand dame" may have acquired an addiction due to her difficulties in coping with the changes concomitant with age. Therefore, behavioral changes secondary to drug intoxication or physiological changes (e.g., circulatory) must always be considered. Themes of loss of family and social supports, fear of or real concerns over physical illnesses, declining physical function and fear of death, and increasing isolation, loneliness, and boredom are found interwoven into many elderly patients' lives.

CASE HISTORY

G. P. is a 69-year-old, white, widowed mother of two grown children. She was admitted from the evaluation unit because of the persistence of feelings of depression which had commenced with the death of her husband one and a half years previously. The patient had been referred to the Center by her family physician for a psychiatric evaluation.

Mrs. P. had been married for nearly fifty years when her husband, while still working full time in his own store, collapsed and died of a coronary thrombosis. Their children subsequently took over the business and remained close to and supportive of their mother. In spite of this, the patient was not able to recover from her husband's death. In the six months prior to admission she had become increasingly seclusive and unstable and felt she could not trust her children, despite their attempts to help her. She began to pester her family physician with incessant complaints of abdominal pain, even though a thorough physical examination and extensive x-ray investigations showed her to be without abdominal pathology. Finally, she confided to the physician that she was afraid that she was going to die of cancer. Since he could do nothing for her, she simply hoped that her demise would occur soon. At this point he decided to refer her to the Center for a psychiatric evaluation.

Mrs. P. was initially seen as an outpatient on the evaluation unit. After a week it became clear that she would need antidepressants, and because of her age it was believed safer to commence such treatment while she was on an inpatient unit; it was also believed that attention could be better focused on solidifying her social supports by the staff.

Following admission, the patient was evaluated both medically and psychologically. A circumscribed history revealed that for the past six weeks she had experienced restless sleep and early morning awakening, and had lost 15 pounds over the past eight weeks. No medical reason could be found which could explain the weight loss, and after a normal EKG tracing was obtained, the patient was commenced on antidepressant medication at lower dose levels than usually used because of her small size and advanced age.

Attention was turned to evaluating her social supports. It was discovered that she lived several miles from either of her children and that much of her previous life had been planned around them and her husband. Her husband's death left her virtually alone save for two friends, both of whom were too infirm to be able to be of any real support. She was isolated, alone, and felt abandoned.

Initially, she rejected the proposal that she live with one of her children—both of whom had the room, the finances to care for her, and the desire to have her live with them—saying, "I will just be a burden like my grandmother was in my parents' home." This, however, appeared to be a moot issue, and the real reason appeared to be related to her sense of finality and fear of irrevocable dependence inherent in the idea of giving up the house she and her husband had lived in for most of their married years and in which they raised their family. The crisis staff focused on these feelings emphasizing the positive support that could be gained by living with her children, where she could be valued for her help in caring for her grandchildren. It was negotiated that she would temporarily move into the home of her oldest daughter where she could have an apartment with her own kitchen and entrance. If this worked out she planned to sell her own home, which meanwhile would have been rented out.

A real drawback to this plan was the fact that Mrs. P. would be leaving her neighborhood and the friends she had known for years. After her mood lifted somewhat, it was ascertained that she had a car and drove it with ease. She was then prevailed upon to take passes from the hospital to visit her friends, who reassured her that they would enjoy having her visit even if she moved out of the neighborhood.

Finally, the patient was helped to find ways to occupy her time after she left the hospital. This process was begun when she was taken to the local volunteer agency by a member of the staff who later talked with her about her marked reluctance to commit herself to any of the jobs. Finally she did decide to spend a few hours a week keeping the books at the family store and also to work as a volunteer at a hospital cafeteria.

On the tenth day of hospitalization the patient was discharged. Her mood was improved, her morbid preoccupation with cancer had disap peared, and she was sleeping through the night. Arrangements were made with her family physician to maintain her on the antidepressants.

Whether it was medication or the social interventions which helped this patient is a moot question. Her case illustrates a number of the typical concerns that elderly patients have. Old age is itself a developmental crisis with an implicit threat and real occurrence of illness, loss, and loneliness. Less fortunate patients also have to contend with major disability, impending death, poverty, and isolation. Sensitive recognition of such problems is imperative for the successful management of these patients, and most respond amazingly well if help is given them in coping with these common stresses.

Crisis of a Chronic Nature

THE RESOURCELESS PATIENT

Occasionally, admission to a crisis unit is precipitated not by a patient's symptoms but by his or her lack of social resources. In such cases the referring agent, such as a social worker, expresses concern at how the person will fare if allowed to remain in the community, given the paucity of social and personal resources at his disposal. In such cases, crisis clinicians find themselves less involved in direct work with the patient than with contacting and negotiating with other agencies on his behalf.

CASE HISTORY

R. P., a 19-year-old, black, Protestant, divorced mother of a two-year-old daughter, was admitted from the emergency room where she had been brought by ambulance after her neighbor saw her have what she described as a seizure. The patient had a history of grand mal epilepsy dating back to age 13, when she was placed on anticonvulsant medication which she had taken up to the present time.

Although little could be learned of the patient's early history, it seemed that she was born in Alabama, the sixth in a family of ten children. She never knew her father, who left her mother shortly after she was born. At age two her mother was pregnant and she was sent to a neighbor whom she continued to live with and who raised her. Her school performance was mediocre, and she began "seeing boys" at age 13 and had intercourse for the first time at age 15. At 17 she became pregnant, and in the third month of her pregnancy she and the boy who had impregnated her were married.

Six months following the birth of a daughter, her husband deserted her and never returned. Her mother then began to care for her child so she could work as a nightclub dancer. She subsequently left this work to come to New Haven with her child and a new lover who in turn left her. She continued living in an apartment, supporting herself with the income from a part-time dancing job.

During the two weeks prior to admission she was robbed twice, losing a television, her money, and some of her clothes. After each robbery she came to the emergency room by ambulance after episodes of epileptic-like behavior. It was after the second episode that she was admitted to the unit.

Upon arrival on the ward the patient appeared alert but pessimistic. She felt that when she was discharged nothing would be changed. Other than a somewhat realistic sense of hopelessness about her situation, her mental status examination was within normal limits. She required no medication other than her usual anticonvulsants.

After a day on the ward, she became friendly with the other patients and through their support and that of the staff began to formulate a plan. She made an appointment at the Division of Vocational Rehabilitation, where job training and counseling were made available to her. Since she felt that returning to her mother would vitiate her attempts toward developing an independent and constructive life for herself, she decided to remain in New Haven and to begin outpatient therapy, with the goal of learning to deal more effectively with her practical problems such as work and the care of her child. During her stay on the crisis unit, she was able to find another woman to share an apartment with.

As part of the information gathering, the records of an earlier neurological work-up had been obtained. Her seizure status was reevaluated, resulting in a readjustment of her medication. Four days after admission she was discharged from the hospital to move into the new apartment with her daughter, who had been staying with a neighbor.

THE RESOURCE-DEVOURING PATIENT

At times, patients present to both inpatient and outpatient units with what appears to be a tolerance to the effects of psychiatric help and social services, much as a narcotic addict becomes tolerant to his drugs. When they initially request help, such patients may evoke sympathy and a desire to assist them, but a scrutiny of the results of past attempts to do so reveals that not only have such efforts not been helpful, but they actually appear to have been detrimental. Such patients seem to do less and less to help themselves the more others help them.

CASE HISTORY

P. D., a 33-year-old, white, separated mother of two children, was admitted because of feelings of depression accompanied by vague suicidal ideation. She was a long-standing member of a methadone maintenance program and visited the Mental Health Center daily for her doses. One of the clinicians associated with the program had noticed her change in mood and initiated her referral to the unit.

The history revealed a chaotic early home life characterized by constant quarrels between her parents over her father's drinking. After his death from cirrhosis when the patient was 16, she began to work in a factory and found an apartment for herself. At 18 she started to experiment with drugs and in two years was using them regularly. At times she prostituted herself in order to obtain the money to support her habit.

At 25 she married a man she had met in a drug treatment program and had two children by him. Their relationship was poor from the beginning, and after both had been hospitalized a number of times for detoxification they separated, although they continued to see each other intermittently.

During the six months preceding admission, it became increasingly apparent that Mrs. D.'s two children were having difficulty at school; the younger one had been referred for a psychiatric evaluation. This had led to a recommendation that he and his mother both visit a child guidance clinic weekly and that he change schools. Mrs. D. became increasingly depressed over the prospect of having to take her son to these appointments and move him to a more distant school. She received public assistance because of her husband's unemployment and, in addition, had a homemaker in twice a week to assist with the housekeeping.

On admission it seemed that the difficulty with her boys was the precipitating stress. She had always been able to cope marginally at best and chronically teetered on the brink of breakdown. This impression was corroborated by information from the agencies which had been assisting her. Additional history from the patient and others suggested that she had been like this for a long time, even preceding the years during which all of the outside resources had been enlisted. It appeared that every time a new service had been added, it resulted in a diminution in her ability to cope. As she put it, "There's something about me that makes people feel sorry for me and want to take care of me." There was no question that she was so overendowed with helping figures that her self-esteem suffered. In addition, her ability to use what personal resources she had was stifled. The focus of the intervention was twofold: to assist her to talk about what it meant to her when everyone involved with her continued to make her feel helpless, and to challenge her to try and change her tactics and become more directed in her own life so as to ward off the ministrations of nearly everyone she came into contact with.

Mrs. D. rose to the occasion and began to mobilize herself rapidly. She herself was able to make arrangements for her son to be taken to and from school each day and worked out how she could get to the child guidance clinic by bus. She obtained employment at a department store, and then was discharged to be followed by the child guidance social worker, to whom we communicated our approach.

THE SOCIOPATHIC PATIENT

Patients with sociopathic character disorders present to mental health centers with the expectation shared by other patients that they too will be helped; however, their demands are not generally those which can be legitimately satisfied by mental health workers. Much difficulty can be avoided in working with these patients if the diagnosis of sociopathy is made early, and the staff alerted to their manipulative behavior patterns. The clearest indicant is a history of antisocial behavior dating to early adolescence.

CASE HISTORY

S. P., a 24-year-old, white, single male, was admitted to the crisis unit from the emergency room because he was believed to be suicidal. The patient told the emergency room clinician that he was feeling hopeless and that he was afraid that he might hurt himself, but could think of no reason why he should feel that way. In the past he had spent several months in jail for minor offenses and had had two brief hospitalizations for "depression."

The patient was raised in the rural South and dropped out of school at age 16 because he stated, "the teachers didn't understand me." His father was an alcoholic but his mother had nonetheless stayed married to him for 30 years. The patient had several encounters with the law prior to entering military service at age 18, but his parents had always assisted him in maneuvering his way out of fines or imprisonment. At age 19 he joined the Army but was discharged after six months because of his constant inability to tolerate authority or regimentation. After discharge he spent a total of six months in prison for assault, petit larceny, and public intoxication. He was unable to maintain any prolonged relationships with a woman but did have sporadic heterosexual affairs. At age 14 he had begun to smoke marijuana and continued to do so intermittently. In addition, he had used mescaline about once a month for the previous year and a half. He denied the use of any other drugs.

The mental status examination was grossly within normal limits. After the initial history had been taken, the patient's mother was interviewed. She revealed that six weeks prior to admission the patient had been arrested for intoxication and had assaulted the arresting officer. For this offense he was scheduled to appear in court. She queried whether it would be possible for us to help her "little boy."

When confronted, Mr. P. vehemently denied that the imminent court appearance was his motive for coming to the hospital, but at the same time he requested a letter to the attorney to be used in court. He was offered a letter documenting that he was in the hospital, a summary of his history, and any other facts his attorney might desire; but he declined this since he doubted that it would be of assistance. He then requested that he be allowed to remain in the hospital until the date of the trial. The staff responded to this by offering to keep him in the hospital only as long as it was felt that he was using the hospitalization constructively to deal with the problems of his likely imprisonment, his low frustration tolerance, and his impoverished interpersonal relationships. After 36 hours of being cajoled into participating in the usual unit routines, the patient left the ward without notifying the staff. He returned home intoxicated several hours later, and his mother called the unit to state that he did not wish to re-enter the hospital.

This case illustrates the limitations of treating such a patient on a crisis ward. Usually, the intervention is confined to evaluation and clarification. To accomplish this one must be extremely conscientious about corroborating all information provided by the patient. It is often necessary to contact family, friends, the police, and any other reliable source because it is easy to be misled by the patient. These patients tend to present themselves in ways which make clinicians want to be sympathetic and make them feel guilty if they do not respond to the patient's demands.

THE CHARACTER DISORDER

Patients with character disorders frequently present on a crisis unit with complaints of how badly the world is treating them and either directly or indirectly request that the hospital help them reestablish a life-long pattern of manipulative behavior that has been rewarding to them in the past. Usually, the hospitalization is the direct result of a breakdown of preexisting behavior patterns that have involved the significant people in the patient's life. Attempts at involving such patients in insight therapy tend to be unrewarding and frustrating. A time-limited mode of therapy is indicated and often proves to be helpful.

Patients with character disorders present a variety of management problems on a crisis unit. No sooner are many of these patients hospitalized than they begin requesting discharge, talking about signing out, and threatening all kinds of mayhem. Others dig in hoping to have their intense dependency needs met by the crisis personnel. Both types of behavior respond best to directness, evenness of temper, and a clear enunciation of what the goals of the crisis unit are. Working with these patients is usually quite taxing on the staff, but can be rewarding, as the following case illustrates.

CASE HISTORY

C. D., a 25-year-old, white, single, unemployed male living at the Y.M.C.A., was admitted to the crisis unit, complaining that he had been depressed "since I lost my job and I think I need to be in the hospital." Three weeks prior to admission, when he was working at a diner, he had accused his employer of being unfair to him in asking him to work on weekends. In anger, he swore at his employer and was fired. Following this episode, his girlfriend of three months broke up with him because, he said, "she was tired of my sponging off her."

For the next few weeks the patient spent hours writing his father long letters in which he described how "sick" he was, how he admired his father, and regretted their inability to be closer during the previous few years. He telephoned his father one evening and told him that he felt he needed to be in a hospital because he was feeling sick and unhappy.

His father drove to the Y.M.C.A. and took him to the emergency room.

C. D. presented on the unit as a shabbily dressed, unshaven, young man who was somewhat taciturn and uncommunicative. He appeared to be sad but was not depressed. In a doleful manner he told us that he "couldn't make it" and that he needed to be looked after.

The patient's early development was essentially normal, but at age 10 he lost his mother to cancer. After her death he became very close to his father. His most pleasant early memory was that of going to football games with his father during the autumn. He did average work in school and had "a lot of friends." Shortly following his 16th birthday, he learned that his father planned to marry a spinster who had diabetes and high blood pressure. Following the marriage, his father paid less attention to him and "used to spend his time taking the old girl from doctor to doctor. She was in and out of hospitals most of the time." The patient's grades plummeted and after his junior year in high school he quit to go to work. From that time on he became involved in a multitude of jobs but never managed to hold one for more than three months. He and his stepmother started to argue interminably, and eventually she told his father that he would have to decide between them, whereupon his father told him that he would have to leave home and fend for himself.

Following his exodus from the home, the patient commenced a pattern of behavior which involved moving from job to job and from city to city. He was usually fired from his jobs following an argument with his employer or a co-worker. He wrote long letters to his father every weekend in which he begged to be allowed to return home. Occasionally, his father sent him money, but the message of his father's letters to him was: "grow up and be a man." Six months prior to his hospitalization, the patient returned to New Haven, arranged to live at the Y.M.-C.A., and found work at the diner. As in the past, he had had no trouble finding women and within a few weeks he started to go steady. His heterosexual relationships, however, were characterized by short-lived exploitative episodes with women who were invariably older than him and who "showed me a good time."

The patient used marijuana occasionally and drank only occasionally. We were not able to elicit a history of a police record or of any misdemeanors. The mental status examination was within normal limits.

The diagnostic impression of C. was of a passive-dependent character disorder whose symptomatology came to the surface around the time of his father's remarriage. He had never resolved his displacement in the home, and it appeared that his need to be sick was a maneuver in which he attempted to reinstate himself in his father's affections, since the latter's taking care of another sick person originally displaced him.

The patient acknowledged that this was true, but no symptomatic improvement or positive motivation resulted. The patient's stepmother refused to come to the hospital, using her physical complaints as an excuse. The patient's father told an interviewer that he realized that C. wanted to come back home and that he would be happy to have him but his wife would not permit it. During the next few days the father tried to influence his wife to change her mind but failed. At this point the patient's father was told that he should try to do whatever he could financially and emotionally for his son. While we recognized that our efforts were playing into C's pathology, it was clear by this stage that no amount of insight, inspiration, or talk would change the patient's attitude. To be of help to him we had to attempt to help him get what he wanted.

The patient's father found a job with an excellent wage for his son and bought him a new suit. He told him that he would do his best to help him out financially. The patient's mood improved considerably, and he became extremely sociable on the unit, at which time he was discharged to outpatient group follow-up.

Psychiatric professionals are often adept at labeling a patient's behavior as manipulative, and having established that they become resistant to allowing or helping the patient achieve what his manipulations are aimed at. This type of response on the part of staff is most appropriate to the application of milieu therapy where the remodeling of a patient's behavior is the goal. But it is counterproductive on a crisis unit. It may be successful in giving the staff the feeling that they are not being manipulated, but unfortunately it often also stands in the way of the patient achieving what may be necessary to keep him out of the hospital.

The Diagnostic Puzzles

THE MEDICAL CASE

At times, patients are admitted to a crisis unit with psychiatric symptoms which turn out to be related directly to a medical illness. On the other hand, "functional" psychiatric illness is frequently accompanied by concurrent physical illness. Crisis clinicians, therefore, must be particularly thorough in evaluation giving attention to the medical history, physical examination, and mental status examination. It is the clinician's responsibility to maintain a high level of suspicion in all cases for causative or coexisting organic illness and to have access to specialist consultation of any type on an emergency basis.

CASE HISTORY

M.T. was a 47-year-old, white, widowed mother of two teenage sons. She was referred to the crisis unit by her internist who had been treating her for "depression" characterized by a 17-pound weight loss over the previous six months, constipation, insomnia characterized by early morning awakening, appetite loss, and suicidal ideation.

The patient first consulted the internist four months prior to hospitalization because she had been weepy, was virtually unable to sleep, and had been dreaming a great deal about her husband when able to sleep; she had lost her husband one year before from lung cancer. Following an unrevealing diagnostic evaluation, including a chest x ray and electrocardiogram, the diagnosis of a "neurotic depression" was made. The patient was given a month's supply of 25 mg Elavil tablets to be taken three times a day and was told to return for monthly reevaluations and prescriptions. Four months of this regimen, however, produced no response, and the internist requested admission for the patient to the crisis unit for further evaluation.

The patient presented as a fully oriented, significantly depressed woman without evidence of a thought or perceptual disorder. On physical examination she appeared cachectic and dehydrated. The initial diagnostic impression was of a depressive neurosis secondary to underlying organic pathology, probably carcinoma. The weight loss, loss of appetite, dehydration, and cachexia pointed strongly to this diagnosis as did the failure to respond to four months of antidepressant medication. Mitigating against this was the fact that the patient had a thorough medical work-up wihtout evidence of pathology and that there were obvious dynamic reasons for a depression—the anniversary of her husband's death. In addition, there was a family history of depression and she herself had experienced a previous depression.

On the evening of her admission, the patient started vomiting, and physical examination revealed a distended abdomen without bowel sounds. She was immediately transferred to a medical unit, where she was found to have a tumor of the lung with large bowel impaction secondary to dehydration. She died two weeks later.

This case demonstrates: 1) that it is important for the psychiatrists who work on a crisis unit to have a solid medical background, so that medical illnesses can be rapidly detected and the appropriate referrals made; 2) that a crisis unit cannot function in isolation, and it is essential that there be a general hospital facility nearby for medical or surgical emergencies.

A DIAGNOSTIC PUZZLE

Occasionally, a patient is referred to the crisis unit for a neuropsychiatric evaluation, either because his diagnosis cannot be readily ascertained by the clinician who is treating him, or because he fails to respond to treatment and it is thought that close observation on an inpatient unit combined with special investigations may add fresh insight. The multidisciplinary approach of the crisis unit provides an opportunity for medical and neuropsychiatric evaluations to be performed by the psychiatric staff using the available consultation facilities, while the nonmedical staff obtains a comprehensive personal and psychiatric history from the patient and from persons intimately involved with him. Information from the latter can sometimes provide a focus for the medical work-up.

CASE HISTORY

D. P., a 28-year-old, white, married father of four children, was referred to the crisis unit by his general practitioner who stated that he had been treating him for schizophrenia and he had shown no response to large doses of a phenothiazine. Mr. P.'s chief complaint was a three-week history of "mental tiredness"; his thought processes were so disorganized that it was impossible to obtain a history from him. A psychiatric nurse interviewed his wife and discovered that he had been well until three weeks prior to admission when he complained of a severe headache which lasted for three days. Following this, she said, he started to become forgetful and confused and to "act strange."

His employer had contacted Mrs. P. and told her that her husband was becoming increasingly forgetful at work and suggested that she take him to the family physician. The physician told her that Mr. P. was in the throes of a "nervous breakdown" and prescribed 40 mg. of perphenazine daily in divided doses. He suggested that Mr. P. continue working and told her to expect a complete recovery within a few days. But instead of improving, Mr. P.'s symptoms grew more severe and he was ultimately referred to the crisis unit.

Mr. P. had a good premorbid adjustment and was a good husband and father. He was a churchgoer, belonged to clubs and community organizations, did not drink, and had never used drugs. There was no history of head injury, loss of consciousness, convulsions, visual difficulty, dizziness, staggering, paralysis, or parasthesia. Physical and neurological examinations were normal. From the case history and mental status examination it was obvious that the patient was suffering from an organic brain syndrome. A lumbar puncture showed 15 lymphocytes per cubic centimeter. C.S.F. protein, sugar, and serology were normal. Skull x rays and a brain scan were normal, but an electroencephalogram demonstrated a slow wave focus. On the basis of these findings the diagnosis of encephalitis was made, and the patient was transferred to a neurological service.

THE UNUSUAL CASE

Hysterical neuroses are encountered infrequently in contemporary society. Occasionally, a patient with such a condition will present or be referred to an emergency room or a psychiatric evaluation service. A brief inpatient hospitalization will often bring about not only a remission of the symptoms but, in addition, the underlying conflicts may be elucidated and resolved, as the following case demonstrates.

CASE HISTORY

U. C., a 28-year-old, white, married mother of two was admitted to the crisis unit from the emergency room following an alleged suicide attempt. It was reported that the patient had been found unconscious in her apartment by a friend, Mrs. Jones, to whom she had recently confided thoughts about suicide. The friend immediately called an ambulance, which took the patient to the emergency room. On arrival the patient was conscious, oriented to time, place, and person, but she seemed somewhat dazed. After she was cleared medically, she informed the psychiatric resident that she had overheard her friend tell the ambulance driver that she had attempted suicide. She stated that, indeed, she had recently entertained thoughts about suicide but said, "A suicide attempt isn't in keeping with my personality. I know myself, and if I were to attempt to kill myself, I'd do it properly."

A comprehensive psychiatric history revealed the patient to be an exceedingly intelligent and successful young woman. Remarkable, however, was the fact that since the eleventh grade she had been involved in a succession of sexual relationships with men and was unable to end one relationship unless another had already commenced. She said that she had recently contemplated leaving her husband, whom "I love very dearly," because she had discovered that he was having an affair.

On the mental status examination the patient appeared dazed and had a global amnesia for the 24 hours prior to her arrival at the emergency room. She was without a thought or perceptual disorder. The diagnostic impression was of a hysterical dissociation with amnesia. A treatment plan was devised in which the patient and her husband would be interviewed seperately and together. The patient expressed a strong desire to recall the events surrounding her discovery in the apartment. She was told that this might occur during the course of the interviews with staff members, but that if it did not, a sodium amytal interview could be performed.

During his interview Mr. C. stated that he had searched the apartment but was unable to find any empty pill bottles. He confirmed that his wife was not the kind of person who would attempt suicide, and he was concerned that something strange had happened to her.

Mrs. Jones, the friend of the patient, was interviewed and said that she had noticed some blood on the patient's panties when she found her but that "the doctors in the emergency room didn't pay any attention to it, and I didn't think it was worth mentioning it at the time." When the patient was told this she responded by saying she believed her husband might have beaten her, as she had threatened to tell his parents about his affair; he had threatened that he would beat her if she did.

For the next two days Mrs. C. continued to be somewhat dazed and unable to recall recent events. She discussed the amytal interview with her husband and a staff member, and requested it because, she stated, "I want this whole business to be cleared up. I don't want there to be any question about my having attempted suicide because that might effect my children should they ever find out. Also, if I was beaten up, I want to know who did it."

During the amytal interview she was able to recount the events of the hours preceding her discovery in the apartment: "When I woke up in the morning I started thinking about the night before when Bill and I argued about his affair and I threatened to go and talk to his parents. I love him too much to do that. I felt trapped. Later on I started to feel numb. I managed to get Bill off to work and the kids off to school. My whole body felt numb. Around noon I went down to the tavern and promised two men there that if they came back to the apartment with me I would sleep with them both. I remember standing in front of the bed in the apartment and I can remember two people in the room with me and their asking me for something and my refusal to do it. Now there's a heavy form on top of me." The patient was not able to recall anything beyond that during the interview.

When interviewed after the amytal had worn off, the patient recounted that she frequently thought that the only way she could break off with Bill would be to be unfaithful to him. She was also able to define the secondary gain involved: "Now perhaps Bill will stop running around and pay more attention to me and the kids." Mr. C., indeed, decided to end his affair and requested referral for psychiatric treatment for himself. Mrs. C. was subsequently discharged to a private psychotherapist.

APPENDIXES

Psychosocial History Forms

NONCOMPUTERIZED FORM

I. Description of the Patient. Age, race, marital status, religion, sex, occupation, legal status (i.e., has he been committed or is he a voluntary admission), residence (where and with whom does he live), source of referral.

II. Chief Complaint.

III. Source(s) of information used in the history.

IV. History of Present Illness. Chronologically describe as accurately as possible (using dates where available) the onset of the patient's acute symptomatology, alterations in behavior, or disturbances of function. Particular attention should be paid to changes in interpersonal relationships, academic or job performance, and extracurricular activities as well as changes in somatic functioning (e.g., sleep disturbance, appetite or weight loss, change in bowel habits, etc.). Mood change and fluctuation is important to document as is use of drugs or medication and where obtained. Suicidal or homicidal ideation should be commented on as well as the presence or absence of such symptoms in the history as hallucinations, derealization, depersonalization, racing thoughts, self-mutilation, paranoid ideation, or ideas of reference. Any change in the patient's recent life situation should be noted (e.g., pregnancy, a death, academic failure, etc.). The patient's previous psychiatric contact (both inpatient and outpatient) should be included in the present illness.

V. Personal History.   The personal history should represent a chronological description of the patient's development and for convenience might be divided into the following sections:

A. **Birth and Early Childhood.**   Was the patient a planned pregnancy or unexpected? Was the patient conceived before marriage? Did the patient's mother have any difficulty before, during, or after the birth? What is the patient's birth order? How long after the previously born sibling or before the next was the patient born? Was the patient's mother depressed after the birth (or suffer other mental disorder)? When did the patient first walk, toilet train, and talk (Or, were they considered "early" or "late")? Was he breast fed or bottle fed? When was he weaned? Did either parent spend a great deal of time away from home early in the patient's life? Did the patient exhibit any childhood symptoms such as head banging, speech disorders, nightmares, bedwetting, phobias, or stuttering? What is the patient's earliest childhood memory?

B. **Family Life.**   Ask the patient to describe his parents, noting whom he talks about first and spends the most time talking about. Did he perceive of them as preferring him or one of his siblings? How does he and how did he perceive the stability of his parents' marriage or their happiness? Did they ever talk of divorce or separation and when? What was his reaction to it? Did he know of either parent having an affair?

C. **Academic Development.**   How old was the patient when he began school? How many years did he go to kindergarten? Did he change schools? Did he attend public, private, or parochial schools? What were his grades like in grade school, junior high school, high school, college, etc.? Was there a dramatic change in his academic performance at any time? What was his major? How far and how old was he when he completed his schooling?

D. **Interpersonal Relationships.**   Trace the patient's quality and quantity of friendships from preschool to the present. How many close friends does he have and how long has he had them? How often does he see his close friends? At any point in his life did he begin to withdraw from others? How many clubs or organizations is he involved in? Has his involvement in groups changed at any point in his life, remote or recent?

E. **Religious Development.** Briefly describe the role religion plays in his life by giving his religion and that of his parents, and to what degree he is involved with the ritual or group functions of his religion.

F. **Psychosexual Development.** Describe the patient's reaction to pubescence (e.g., growth of facial hair, onset of menses, breast development). Who first explained sex to the patient? Does he masturbate or has he in the past, and how does he feel about it? When did he begin to date, neck and pet, have intercourse? Has he had many sexual partners? When was his first sustained long-term relationship? Was the patient ever engaged or married? Is he married now? How long did he court his wife? If divorced, give circumstances of divorce both as perceived by patient and as legally defined (e.g., mental cruelty). How is his sexual adjustment? How frequently does he have intercourse? Is it enjoyable? If a woman, ask about the periodicity of her menses and her reaction to them. What mode of contraception do they use? How many children do they have, and how did they respond to pregnancy? Have either had any extramarital affairs? How is the marriage going at present and what are the future plans? Has the patient ever had any homosexual experience? Has the patient ever had an abortion or miscarriage? If an older woman, when was the patient's menopause and how did she respond to it?

G. **Occupational History.** What is the patient's present occupation and how long has he been employed? Has there been any change in his work situation (e.g., promotion, transfer to another area)? How many jobs has the patient had and how long has he held them? What were the circumstances of any change of occupation? What are his sources of income and are they adequate?

H. **Housing History.** Where and with whom does the patient live? Has he moved recently? Where else has he lived and what were the circumstances of moving?

I. **Family History.** If the patient's parents are living, note their age, health, occupation, and place of residence—also any divorce and remarriage. If either or both parents are dead, inquire about the time and cause of death. Ask the same questions relevant to age, occupation, education, health, and residence of the patient's siblings, spouse, and children. Specifically, inquire into a family history of mental illness (ask about "depression"), neurological disease, alcoholism, epilepsy, and mental retardation.

J. **Medical History.**   Inquire into the person's past and present history of medical illnesses, operations, trauma, and hospitalizations.

K. **Drug Use History.**   Is the patient taking any medication? What is and has been his alcoholic consumption? Is there any change? Is he addicted to any drugs (e.g., heroin, barbiturates)? Does he or has he used amphetamines (e.g., "speed"), hallucinogens (e.g., LSD, mescaline, psilocybin, STP, DMT), or marijuana? If so, how frequently and what is his reaction to it?

L. **Military History.**   What is the patient's military status? If discharged from the service, what were the circumstances of discharge?

M.**Legal History.**   Has the patient ever been imprisoned for any offenses? Is there legal action pending?

COMPUTERIZED FORM*

*Psychiatric Anamnestic Record (Form MS O4) Reproduced by permission of Robert L. Spitzer, M.D. and Jean Endicott, Ph.D.

Form MS 04
PSYCHIATRIC ANAMNESTIC RECORD (PAR)*   Read instructions on reverse side.

Patient's last name	First name	M.I.	Facility	Ward

IDENTIFICATION
Case or consecutive number

=0= =1= =2= =3= =4=   =5= =6= =7= =8= =9=
=0= =1= =2= =3= =4=   =5= =6= =7= =8= =9=
=0= =1= =2= =3= =4=   =5= =6= =7= =8= =9=
=0= =1= =2= =3= =4=   =5= =6= =7= =8= =9=
=0= =1= =2= =3= =4=   =5= =6= =7= =8= =9=

Facility code

=0= =1= =2= =3= =4=   =5= =6= =7= =8= =9=
=0= =1= =2= =3= =4=   =5= =6= =7= =8= =9=
=0= =1= =2= =3= =4=   =5= =6= =7= =8= =9=

Rater code

=0= =1= =2= =3= =4=   =5= =6= =7= =8= =9=
=0= =1= =2= =3= =4=   =5= =6= =7= =8= =9=
=0= =1= =2= =3= =4=   =5= =6= =7= =8= =9=

Date of admission to facility

	Jan	Feb	Mar	Apr	May	Month	Jun	Jul	Aug	Sep	Oct
	1	69	70	71	72	Year	73	74	75	Nov	Dec
	2	3	4	5	6		7	8	9	10	11
	12	13	14	15	16	Day	17	18	19	20	21
	22	23	24	25	26		27	28	29	30	31

Status on admission   inpatient day night OPD other

TRANSACTION
first admission   re-admission   correction   deletion

DESCRIPTION
Sex   male   female

Ethnic group   ?   White   Negro Puerto Rican Oriental Amer Indian Other

Age
=0= =1= =2= =3= =4=   =5= =6= =7= =8= =9=
=0= =1= =2= =3= =4=   =5= =6= =7= =8= =9=

Marital status   married divorced widowed separated annulled never married

Siblings (living or dead) is a twin   other multiple births

0   1   2   3   4   5   6   7   8   9+

ATTITUDE TOWARDS ADMISSION
?   positive   neutral   ambivalent   negative   very negative

INFORMANTS

physician	nonmedical therapist	school
patient	family member	friend
associate	other facility or agency	police

*Developed by Robert L. Spitzer, M.D. and Jean Endicott, Ph.D., Biometrics Research, N.Y.S. Department of Mental Hygiene, with the assistance of the Multi-State Information System for Psychiatric Patients Project. Supported by N.Y.S. Department of Mental Hygiene, C29820 and NIMH Grants 14934 and 08534.

IBM M65 1997

RELIABILITY AND COMPLETENESS OF INFORMATION
?   very good   good   only fair   poor   very poor

CHARACTERISTICS OF CURRENT CONDITION
exacerbation of chronic condition   recurrence of similar previous condition

indistinguishable from past   significant change from any previous condition

Onset of current condition   sudden   gradual   very gradual

Duration of current condition
Unit   days   weeks   months   years

=0= =1= =2= =3= =4=   =5= =6= =7= =8= =9=
=0= =1= =2= =3= =4=   =5= =6= =7= =8= =9=

Precipitating stress   ?   none   slight   mild   mod   mark

drug reaction	traumatic incident	someone's death
financial	physical illness in family	physical illness in patient
sexual problems	family problems	nonfamily interpersonal problems
school problems	occupational problems	other change in life circumstances

→ Course since onset of current condition
worsened greatly   worsened somewhat   remained stable   variable   improved somewhat   greatly improved

PSYCHIATRIC DISTURBANCE IN FAMILY
functional psych illness   organic brain syndrome

Mother   ?   none | mild   severe   mild   severe
Father   ?   none | mild   severe   mild   severe
→ Siblings at least mildly ill   ?   1   2   3   4+

PREVIOUS TREATMENT FOR PSYCHIATRIC DISTURBANCE   ? none → next section

Age when first treated (any treatment)
=0= =1= =2= =3= =4=   =5= =6= =7= =8= =9=
=0= =1= =2= =3= =4=   =5= =6= =7= =8= =9=

Treated at (all occasions)   residential treatment   rehabilitation facility   educat special classes   outpatient Rx   partial hosp   psychiatric hospitalization (not including this one)

→ number   1   2   3   4   5   6   7   8+

Age at first hospitalization (not including this one)
=0= =1= =2= =3= =4=   =5= =6= =7= =8= =9=

=0= =1= =2= =3= =4=   =5= =6= =7= =8= =9=

Total time of psychiatric hospitalizations (not including this one)
Unit   days   weeks   months   years

=0= =1= =2= =3= =4=   =5= =6= =7= =8= =9=
=0= =1= =2= =3= =4=   =5= =6= =7= =8= =9=

Set no. 0074187   Mark last 3 digits of Set number in area below

=0= =1= =2= =3= =4=   =5= =6= =7= =8= =9=
=0= =1= =2= =3= =4=   =5= =6= =7= =8= =9=
=0= =1= =2= =3= =4=   =5= =6= =7= =8= =9=

PAR 1b

PURPOSE
The purpose of the Psychiatric Anamnestic Record (PAR) is to enable a rater to record the information pertinent to a patient's psychiatric anamnesis. Proper use of this form encourages the rater to seek information on all of the items on the PAR when obtaining a history. The recorded information can be used by a computer to produce a narrative account of the patient's psychiatric history. In addition, it will also be possible to use the information for the systematic evaluation of individual patients and for studies of groups of patients.

The rater may add to the clinical record narrative comments for any information for which there are no items on the form.

DATA SOURCE
The data upon which the judgments are based should be from any reliable source: the patient himself, reports of family or friends, past hospital or clinic records or letters of referral.

TIME PERIOD
The time period for items varies. The specific time period to be considered (e.g. last month, age 12 up to last month, last 5 years) is noted either within the item or at the beginning of an entire section.

ITEMS OF INFORMATION
Some items must be marked for all patients. These items are printed in **bold**. For example:

Suicidal gestures

All of the remaining items are marked only when applicable to the patient being evaluated and when sufficient information is available. Example:

Depressed mood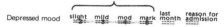

When an item requires a scaled judgment, (where the rater selects the most appropriate term from a list of terms) these terms are linked by a shaded line. All other items are true-false, and as many as are true should be noted.

All scaled judgments of severity should take into account how intense the behavior was as well as how much of the time it was present during the period under study. Thus, the ratings are a weighted average for the entire time period and not necessarily the highest intensity exhibited at any one point in time. When making these judgments, the rater should think of the full range of the behavior that people sometimes exhibit.

NOTING JUDGMENTS
Note all judgments with a No. 2 pencil. Make a heavy dark mark between the lines of the grids. Example: ▬ To change a judgment, completely erase the incorrect mark. In filling out IDENTIFICATION section and Set number, numbers should be written in the boxes as well as noted in the grids. The numbers read from top to bottom so that the last digit is in the bottom row. If the number has fewer digits than the number of rows allotted, one or more of the top rows are left blank.

PRINTOUT
The computer printout will contain in a narrative all of the information that the rater has noted. This will include information based on ratings of "none" as well as positive indications of psychopathology.

If a rater fails to mark an item that is supposed to be completed for all patients, the printout will note that information for this item is missing.

DEFINITIONS AND INSTRUCTIONS for sections and items which may be unclear.

IDENTIFICATION
Rater code Code number for person completing this form.

TRANSACTION
For all transactions, all four pages must be submitted.
First admission for subject to this facility.
Readmission of this subject to this facility.
Correction Entry of IDENTIFICATION and one or more sections of the form to indicate new information or a clerical or judgmental error in the information for those sections of a previous form. The sections must contain all relevant data since the information submitted on the form will completely replace what was in the record for those sections. The IDENTIFICATION section must be identical to the previous entry.
Deletion Erasure of entire record for date noted. Only IDENTIFICATION should be completed. Example: Record to be deleted was for another patient or had the wrong date.

ATTITUDE TOWARDS ADMISSION
If the patient is now being treated in an institution or some other facility, note his attitude towards admission.
Unknown As might be the case with a mute patient.
Ambivalent At times positive, at other times, negative.
Neutral No particular emotional reaction.

RELIABILITY AND COMPLETENESS OF INFORMATION
Rater's overall judgment of accuracy and completeness of information. Example: a mute catatonic would not give information about the content of his thoughts, thereby lowering the completeness of the overall information.

CHARACTERISTICS OF CURRENT CONDITION
Note that more than one of these four items may be used to describe the current condition.
Exacerbation of chronic condition A worsening of a long standing condition.
Recurrence of similar previous condition Symptomatology of present condition resembles that of a previous episode.
Indistinguishable from past Current condition is essentially a continuation of a long standing past condition without noticeable change in symptomatology.
Significant change from any previous condition Symptomatology differs markedly from any previous symptomatology demonstrated by patient.

Duration of current condition If the current condition is judged to be an exacerbation of a chronic condition, the duration should be from the onset of the exacerbation.

Note duration in terms of either days, weeks, months or years with the appropriate number. The possible range is "one day" to "more than fifteen years."

Precipitating stress which is judged to be related to onset of current condition. Severity of stress is in terms of what a normal person's reaction would most likely be if he were in a comparable situation. If severity is "slight" or more, note the nature of stresses.

PSYCHIATRIC DISTURBANCE IN FAMILY
Note presence or history of psychiatric disturbance in natural family members, whether treated or not.

PREVIOUS TREATMENT FOR PSYCHIATRIC DISTURBANCE
Consider the six categories listed.
Treated at
    Special education classes for the retarded or emotionally disturbed.
    Outpatient therapy All treatment by persons with specialized training for a disturbance in subject's mood, thinking or behavior given in an outpatient setting.
    Partial hospitalization Day, night, or weekend care.
    Rehabilitation facility where special training is given.
    Psychiatric hospitalization 24 hour inpatient care. Include psychiatric care in a general hospital. Do not count direct transfers between hospitals as separate admissions.

SET NUMBER
Page one of each PAR is preprinted with a seven digit Set number. The last three digits of this number are used to link the four pages together for data processing. Be sure to mark the last three digits from the Set number on all four pages.

IBM M61998

PREVIOUS TREATMENT (continued)

Treatments received (as outpatient or inpatient)   ?

		indiv supportive psychotherapy
drugs	counseling	
indiv dynamic psychotherapy	group psychotherapy	behavior therapy
ECT	brain surgery	insulin coma
family psychotherapy	vocational rehabilitation	hypnosis

Most likely diagnosis of condition(s) treated previously   ?

mental retardation	organic brain syndrome	schizophrenia
psychotic affective disorder	neurosis	antisocial personality
other personality disorder	sexual deviation	alcoholism
drug dependence	psychophysiologic disorder	transient sit disorder
behavior disorder of childhood & adolescence	condition without manifest psychiatric disorder	non-specific condition

CHILDHOOD (prior to age 12)

Problems   ?   no apparent problems

withdrawn	hallucinations	bizarre behavior
enuresis	school phobia	excessive fears
temper tantrums	stuttering	extreme shyness
excessive agression	destructiveness	fire setting
stealing	sadism	chronic lying
no friends	school truancy	hyperactivity

Raised by (all that apply)

both natural parents	one natural parent	other relatives
foster parents	adoptive parents	insti- tution

Adequacy of environment for personality development

?	very good	good	fair	poor	very poor

ADOLESCENT FRIENDSHIP PATTERN (12-18)

Relationship with friends	?	no friends	or	very good	good	only fair	poor	very poor
Good friends	many	several		a few	only one	none	preferred being alone
avoided groups		enjoyed group activities				was a leader	

ADULT FRIENDSHIP PATTERN (last 5 years)   not adult → skip section

Relationship with friends	?	no friends	or	very good	good	only fair	poor	very poor
Good friends	many	several		a few	only one	none	preferred being alone
avoided groups		enjoyed group activities				was a leader	

EDUCATION AND INTELLECTUAL CAPACITY

Education (level completed)
completed grade

?	none	1-5	6	7	8	high school 9	10	11	12

college or business school less 1 1yr	2yr	3yr	4yr	some graduate school	graduate school degree

Overall academic performance (junior high and beyond)

?	super- ior	very good	aver- age	only fair	poor	very poor	vari- able	consis- tent

Estimate of intellectual capacity

?	superior	bright	average	borderline	retarded

OCCUPATIONAL HISTORY
Highest occupational level ever attained

?	never worked	higher executive	proprietor large business	major professional
business manager	proprietor medium business	lesser professional	owner small business
administrative personnel	large farm owner	semi- professional	clerical worker
sales worker	technician	owner little business	farm owner
small farm owner	skilled manual employee	semiskilled employee	unskilled employee

During last 5 years was employed (for pay)

?	virtually all time	almost all time	most of time	about half	less than half	only briefly	not at all

at (predominantly)	full time job	half time job	less than half time

Amount of time employed during last 5 years limited by   retirement

		going to school
physical illness	psycho- pathology	
household responsibilities	type of work	job market

Work performance last 5 years (if worked at all)

?	superior	very good	good	aver- age	only fair	poor	very poor

Change in occupational status or responsibility last 5 years (if worked)

?	marked elevation	some elevation	no change	some decline	marked decline

ADOLESCENT HETEROSEXUAL ADJUSTMENT

Overall	?	excel- lent	very good	good	fair	poor	very poor
Sexual activity	none	little	average	excessive			
Dated	rarely	occa- sionally	often	Sexual curiosity	little	none	
Promiscuous	occa- sionally	often					

HIGHEST LEVEL ADULT HETEROSEXUAL ADJUSTMENT OVER A SUSTAINED PERIOD   not adult → skip sect

Overall	?	excel- lent	very good	good	fair	poor	very poor
Sexual activity	none	little	average	excessive			
Impotent	often	usually	occa- sionally	Premature ejaculation	often	usu- ally	
Promiscuous	occa- sionally	often		Frigid	often	usu- ally	

SEXUAL DEVIATIONS

							relation to partners
Homosexual activity							
Adolescent	?	none	rare	occa- sional	fre- quent	very freq	ca- sual friends
Adult	?	none	rare	occa- sional	fre- quent	very freq	ca- sual friends
Other deviations as adult				exhibitionism	voyeurism	trans- vestism	

MARRIAGE   never married → skip section

If married more than once, number

		2	3	4	5+

reason(s):	divorced	annulled
death	bigamy	

Set no.   Mark last 3 digits of Set number from page 1.

:=0:	::1:	::2:	::3:	::4:		::5:	::6:	::7:	::8:	::9:
:=0:	::1:	::2:	::3:	::4:		::5:	::6:	::7:	::8:	::9:
:=0:	::1:	::2:	::3:	::4:		::5:	::6:	::7:	::8:	::9:

IBM M6 1999

PAR 2b

Most likely diagnosis or diagnoses of condition(s) treated previously Use American Psychiatric Association's Diagnostic and Statistical Manual, Second Edition, 1968, for descriptions.

CHILDHOOD
Problems

Withdrawn Avoidance of contact or involvement with others.

Hallucinations Sensory perceptions in the absence of identifiable stimulation.

Bizarre behavior Behavior that is odd or eccentric.

Enuresis Inappropriate and involuntary passage of urine after the age when bladder control is expected.

School phobia Refusal to attend school because of an irrational fear.

Stuttering Spasmodic speaking with involuntary pauses and repetitions.

Extreme shyness Extreme discomfort with people.

Excessive aggression Fighting, bullying to an excessive degree.

Destructiveness Destroying his own or other people's property.

Sadism Enjoyment from inflicting physical or psychological pain on animals or people.

School truancy Nonattendance at school for reasons other than school phobia.

Hyperactivity Excessive restlessness and overactivity.

Adequacy of environment for personality development Consider all aspects of family and community environment including emotional climate of family, poverty, and community problems.

ADOLESCENT FRIENDSHIP PATTERN
Relationship with friends Consider intimacy, continuity, pleasure derived, and degree of ambivalence or destructiveness.

Estimate of intellectual capacity Take into account ingenuity, and creativity, as well as vocabulary and academic achievements. Superior: IQ 120+, Bright: 110-119, Average: 90-109, Borderline: 70-89, Retarded: below 70.

OCCUPATIONAL HISTORY
Examples of occupations at various levels

Higher executive in government or large businesses, military officer (major or above).

Proprietor large business worth over $100,000.

Major professional accountant (CPA), chemist, clergyman (trained), teacher (college), physician, lawyer.

Business manager advertising director, brokerage salesman, minor government official, office manager, police chief, personnel manager.

Proprietor medium business worth $35,000-$100,000.

Lesser professional librarian, musician (symphony), R.N., social worker, teacher (elementary or high school), engineer (no degree).

Owner small business worth $6,000-$35,000.

Administrative personnel chief clerk, insurance agent, private secretary, service manager, sales representative.

Large farm owner of farm worth $20,000-$35,000.

Semi-professional actor, clergyman (not trained), commercial artist, laboratory assistant, mortician, photographer, reporter

Clerical worker bank teller, business machine operator, employment interviewer, railroad conductor.

Sales worker sales clerk in store.

Technician draftsman, inspector, maintenance supervisor, proofreader, switchboard operator.

Owner little business worth $3,000-$6,000.

Farm owner of farm worth $10,000-$20,000.

Small farm owner farm tenant who owns farm equipment.

Skilled manual employee butcher, carpenter, electrician, fireman, hair stylist, mason, plumber, policeman, repairman, printer.

Semi-skilled employee hospital aide, bus driver, dressmaker, elevator operator, enlisted man, factory machine operator, guard, short order cook.

Unskilled employee attendant, counterman, domestic, farm helper, laborer, peddler, stagehand.

Amount of time employed during last five years limited by Include both limitation on hours per week as well as portion of five years employed at all.

Work performance Consider frequent job changes because of his attitude or behavior, how well he performed the duties of the job, and how satisfied others were with his work or behavior.

Change in occupational status or responsibility during time employed Consider promotions, job titles, recognition, and amount of supervision of self or others. Do not consider automatic salary increases

ADOLESCENT HETEROSEXUAL ADJUSTMENT
Overall Take into account dating, sexual curiosity, sexual activity, and comfort in heterosexual activities.

Promiscuous Sexual relations with numerous partners without emotional intimacy.

HIGHEST LEVEL OF ADULT HETEROSEXUAL ADJUSTMENT OVER A SUSTAINED PERIOD
The items in this section all refer to the patient's highest level of functioning for a period of at least 6 months. For example, a 55 year old man who in his thirties had good heterosexual adjustment, would be given that rating even if he had poor adjustment during his later years.

Overall Consider sexual performance and satisfaction, and emotional intimacy with partners.

Premature ejaculation Ejaculation so quickly that partner cannot be satisfied.

Impotent Difficulty maintaining an erection during intercourse.

Frigid Psychogenically inhibited female sexual response.

SEXUAL DEVIATIONS
Homosexuality Overt sexual relations between members of the same sex.

Exhibitionism Inappropriate exposure of genitals.

Voyeurism Compulsive interest in observing sexual activity or genitals of other people.

Transvestism Sexual pleasure from dressing in the clothing of the opposite sex.

MARRIAGE (continued)

Age when first married ___?___

::1:: ::2:: ::3:: ::4::   ::5:: ::6:: ::7:: ::8:: ::9::

::0:: ::1:: ::2:: ::3:: ::4::   ::5:: ::6:: ::7:: ::8:: ::9::

Marital adjustment (if currently married)

	very good	good	only fair	poor	very poor

NUMBER OF OWN CHILDREN

	0	1	2	3	4	5	6	7+
Alive								
Dead	0	1	2	3	4	5	6	7+

PHYSICAL HEALTH

	?	very good	good	only fair	poor	very poor
Up to age 12						
After age 12	?	very good	good	only fair	poor	very poor

Permanent brain damage — suspected / likely / definite

beginning at — prenatal period / birth / childhood / adolescence / adulthood

Seizures occurred — prior to age 12 / age 12 to last month / last month

SIGNS AND SYMPTOMS SINCE AGE 12

Impaired relations with :	age 12 to last month slight	mild	mod	mark	last month	reason for admission
parents					:LM:	:RA:
associates					:LM:	:RA:
boyfriend(s)					:LM:	:RA:
girlfriend(s)					:LM:	:RA:
spouse					:LM:	:RA:
children					:LM:	:RA:

Impaired performance at:

		last month	reason for admission
school	(covered previously)	:LM:	:RA:
job	(covered previously)	:LM:	:RA:
housekeeping		:LM:	:RA:

Delusions	?	absent	suspected	likely	definite	:LM:	:RA:
		slight	mild	mod	mark		
persecutory						:LM:	:RA:
somatic						:LM:	:RA:
grandeur						:LM:	:RA:
guilt						:LM:	:RA:
religious						:LM:	:RA:
influence						:LM:	:RA:
nihilistic						:LM:	:RA:

Hallucinations	?	absent	suspected	likely	definite	:LM:	:RA:
		slight	mild	mod	mark		
auditory						:LM:	:RA:
visual						:LM:	:RA:
olfactory						:LM:	:RA:
gustatory						:LM:	:RA:
tactile						:LM:	:RA:
visceral						:LM:	:RA:

SIGNS AND SYMPTOMS SINCE AGE 12 (continued)

	age 12 to last month slight	mild	mod	mark	last month	reason for admission
Depressed mood					:LM:	:RA:
Anxiety					:LM:	:RA:
Poor appetite					:LM:	:RA:
Insomnia					:LM:	:RA:
Phobia(s)					:LM:	:RA:
Obsession(s)					:LM:	:RA:
Compulsion(s)					:LM:	:RA:
Guilt					:LM:	:RA:
Broods excessively					:LM:	:RA:
Excessive anger					:LM:	:RA:
Antisocial behavior					:LM:	:RA:
Autistic thinking					:LM:	:RA:
Grandiosity					:LM:	:RA:
Assaultive					:LM:	:RA:
Suspiciousness					:LM:	:RA:
Unwarranted concern with physical health					:LM:	:RA:
Psychophysiologic reactions					:LM:	:RA:
Easily fatigued					:LM:	:RA:
Homosexual fears					:LM:	:RA:
Sexual deviations	(covered previously)				:LM:	:RA:
Impaired sexual functioning					:LM:	:RA:
Withdrawal					:LM:	:RA:
Disorientation					:LM:	:RA:
Inappropriate behavior					:LM:	:RA:
Apathy					:LM:	:RA:
Dissociative symptoms					:LM:	:RA:
Depersonalization					:LM:	:RA:
Conversion reactions					:LM:	:RA:
Impaired memory					:LM:	:RA:
Disorganized speech					:LM:	:RA:
Psychomotor retardation					:LM:	:RA:
Psychomotor excitement					:LM:	:RA:
Impaired functioning goal directed activities					:LM:	:RA:

Set no. Mark last 3 digits of Set number from page 1.

::0:: ::1:: ::2:: ::3:: ::4:: [ ] ::5:: ::6:: ::7:: ::8:: ::9::

::0:: ::1:: ::2:: ::3:: ::4:: [ ] ::5:: ::6:: ::7:: ::8:: ::9::

::0:: ::1:: ::2:: ::3:: ::4:: [ ] ::5:: ::6:: ::7:: ::8:: ::9::

IBM M62001

PAR 3b

MARRIAGE
Marital adjustment Consider all aspects of marital relationship.

PHYSICAL HEALTH
Consider seriousness of conditions and chronicity.
Permanent brain damage Include all forms of chronic organic brain syndrome as well as motor or sensory dysfunction resulting from permanent brain tissue damage.
Prenatal period Examples: retardation associated with maternal infection with Rubella, Down's syndrome.
Birth Example: anoxia during delivery.

SIGNS AND SYMPTOMS SINCE AGE 12
In this section, all of the items can be rated in three different ways: severity from age 12 to last month, as present during the last month, and as a reason for this admission. To be meaningful, only a relatively few items should be noted as a reason for admission. In almost all cases, items noted as a reason for admission will also have been noted as present during the last month.

Items marked as reason for admission (in this section as well as in the next section, PERSONALITY TRAITS), will be grouped together on the computer printout.

Impaired relations with Include all difficulties caused by patient's own behavior attitude, or feelings.

Delusions Conviction in some important personal belief which is almost certainly not true. Note type if suspected, likely, or definite.
Persecutory delusions Examples: believes an organized conspiracy exists against him, or that he has been attacked, harassed, cheated or persecuted or that people talk about him or stare at him, when the circumstances make it almost certainly not true.
Somatic delusions Conviction about his body that is almost certainly not true, e.g. body is rotting, someone is in his brain.
Delusions of grandeur Claims power or knowledge beyond the bounds of credibility, e.g. has special relation to God; can read people's minds.
Delusions of guilt Belief that he has done something terrible or is responsible for some event or condition which is almost certainly not true, e.g. has ruined family by his bad thoughts.
Religious delusions A delusion involving a religious theme.
Delusions of influence Claims his thoughts, mood, or actions are controlled or mysteriously influenced by other people or by strange forces.
Nihilistic delusions Believes the world is destroyed or that he or everyone is dead.

Hallucinations Sensory perceptions in the absence of identifiable stimulation occurring during the waking state whether judged to be on an organic, functional psychotic, or hysterical basis. Note type if suspected, likely, or definite.
Auditory hallucinations Hallucinations of sounds.
Visual hallucinations Hallucinations of visual images.
Olfactory hallucinations Hallucinations of smell.
Gustatory hallucinations Hallucinations of taste.
Tactile hallucinations Hallucinations of touch.
Visceral hallucinations Hallucinations of sensations arising within the body.

Depression Sadness, worthlessness, failure, hopelessness, remorse, or loss.
Anxiety Apprehension, worry, nervousness, tension, fearfulness, or panic.
Insomnia Difficulty falling or staying asleep.
Phobia Irrational fear of a specific object or situation, e.g. fear of crowds, heights, animals; to be distinguished from free floating anxiety or fears of general conditions (getting sick, business failure).
Obsession Persistent, unwanted thoughts which occur against his resistance, the content of which he regards as senseless, e.g. thoughts of killing child.
Compulsion An insistent, repetitive, unwanted urge to perform an act which is contrary to his ordinary conscious wishes or standards, e.g. hand washing compulsion.
Broods excessively Excessive preoccupation with unpleasant thoughts or feelings.

Excessive anger Anger which is disproportionate to the situation.
Antisocial behavior Examples: lying, stealing, cheating.
Autistic thinking Thinking which is egocentric and illogical, in which objective facts tend to be obscured, distorted, or excluded.
Grandiosity Inflated appraisal of his worth, contact, power or knowledge.
Assaultive Physical violence directed toward some other person.
Suspicious From mild distrust to feelings of persecution not warranted by actual situation.
Unwarranted concern with physical health Concern with physical health that is apparently not warranted by actual physical condition. Include concern with one organ (e.g. cardiac neurosis) as well as with multiple organs (hypochondriasis).
Psychophysiologic reactions Physical symptoms usually mediated by the autonomic nervous system, and clearly caused by emotional factors. The physiological changes are those that normally accompany certain emotional states, are generally reversable and therefore do not involve permanent tissue alteration.
Homosexual fears Irrational fear that he is or will become a homosexual or that he will be homosexually attacked.
Impaired sexual functioning Consider sexual functioning in the context of age appropriate activities.
Withdrawal Avoidance of contact or involvement with people.
Disorientation Loss of awareness of the position of the self in relation to time, place and other persons.
Inappropriate Behavior that is odd, eccentric or not in keeping with the situation. Examples: exposing self, talking to self, frequent giggling.
Apathy Lack of feeling, interest, concern or emotion.
Dissociation A psychological separation or splitting off of behavior or events from consciousness. Examples: trance, amnesia, fugue, hysterical attack, somnambulism.
Depersonalization Feelings of strangeness or unreality about one's own body, e.g. feels outside of body or as if part of body does not belong to him.
Conversion reaction A disturbance of the special senses or of the voluntary motor system, often expressing emotional conflict in a symbolic manner; to be distinguished from psychophysiologic disorders which are mediated by the autonomic nervous system, from malingering which is done consciously, and from neurological lesions which cause anatomically circumscribed symptoms.
Disorganized speech Impairment in the form of speech which makes it difficult to follow or understand. When severe, speech is incoherent.
Psychomotor retardation Generalized slowing down of physical reactions and movements.
Psychomotor excitement Generalized overactivity.
Impaired functioning in goal directed activities Include impaired efficiency or effectiveness in carrying out tasks or activities which he or others expect him to complete. Examples: job, daily routine, leisure time activities.

IBM M62002

SIGNS AND SYMPTOMS SINCE AGE 12 (continued)

Excessive use of	Age 12 to last month				last month	reason for admission
	slight	mild	mod	mark		
alcohol	2	3	4	5	M	RA
narcotics	2	3	4	5	M	RA
barbiturates	2	3	4	5	M	RA
stimulants	2	3	4	5	M	RA
hallucinogens	2	3	4	5	M	RA
cannabis	2	3	4	5	M	RA
other substances	2	3	4	5	M	RA
Suicidal preoccupation	2	3	4	5	M	RA

	?	never	once	several	many		
Suicidal gestures		never	once	several	many	M	RA
Suicidal attempts	?	never	once	several	many	M	RA

PERSONALITY TRAITS (not limited to episodes of illness)

	slight	mild	mod	mark		
Rigid		3	4	5		RA
Inhibited	2	3	4	5		RA
Unable to relax	2	3	4	5		RA
Overly conscientious	2	3	4	5		RA
Emotionally distant	2	3	4	5		RA
Emotionally unstable	2	3	4	5		RA
Excitable	2	3	4	5		RA
Histrionic	2	3	4	5		RA
Cyclothymic (mood swings)	2	3	4	5		RA
Impulsive	2	3	4	5		RA
Stubborn	2	3	4	5		RA
Passive-aggressive	2	3	4	5		RA
Self-defeating	2	3	4	5		RA
Dependent	2	3	4	5		RA
Aimless	2	3	4	5		RA
Hostile (overt)	2	3	4	5		RA
Suspicious	2	3	4	5		RA
Domineering	2	3	4	5		RA
Eccentric	2	3	4	5		RA
Hypersensitive (to others)	2	3	4	5		RA
Tending to blame others	2	3	4	5		RA

Traits which may be positive or negative

	?	pract none	little	only fair	mod-erate	consid-erable
Pleasure out of life		pract none	little	only fair	mod-erate	consid-erable
Involvement in voluntary leisure time activities		pract none	little	only fair	mod-erate	consid-erable
		very poor	poor	only fair	good	very good
Sense of humor						

PERSONALITY TRAITS (continued)

	very irresponsible	somewhat irresponsible	generally responsible	very responsible
Responsible				
	pract none	little	only fair	aver-age	consid-erable
Concern for others					
	very poor	poor	only fair	aver-age	consid-erable
Ability to cope with stress					
	very poor	poor	only fair	good	very good
Judgment					
	pract none	little	mod-erate	a great deal
Ambitious				
	pract none	little	mod-erate	a great deal
Perseverance				

ARRESTS

never

Number	?	1	2	3	4	5	6	7+

For	assault	fraud	theft
disorderly conduct	sexual offense	reckless driving	
murder	drug possession	illegal gambling	

Convictions	1	2	3	4	5	6	7+

Punishments	suspended sentence	prison	fine

PREVIOUS EPISODES

no episodes

Number (all kinds) of previous episodes (best guess)

?	1	2	3	4	5	6	7	8	9+

Number of previous episodes lasting more than one week where depression or elation of at least moderate intensity was predominant.

?	1	2	3	4	5	6	7	8	9+

Episodes	all elated	all depressed	depressed and elated

OVERALL SEVERITY OF ILLNESS

Prior to age 12

?	not ill	slight	mild	mod	mark	severe	among most extre	was overtly psychotic

Age 12 to last month

?	not ill	slight	mild	mod	mark	severe	among most extre	was overtly psychotic

Last month

?	not ill	slight	mild	mod	mark	severe	among most extre	was overtly psychotic

Age when first demonstrated significant impairment because of psychopathology   ?   never

0	1	2	3	4	5	6	7	8	9
0	1	2	3	4	5	6	7	8	9

RATER HAS WRITTEN COMMENTS ELSEWHERE

Signature	Date

Set no. Mark last 3 digits of Set number from page 1.

0	1	2	3	4		5	6	7	8	9
0	1	2	3	4		5	6	7	8	9
0	1	2	3	4		5	6	7	8	9

PAR 4b

Excessive use of Consider psychological or physiological dependence, and interference with performance of daily routine or expected duties.

Narcotics Demerol, Morphine, Cocaine, Heroin.
Barbiturates Seconal, Nembutal, Phenobarbital.
Stimulants Dexedrine, Amphetamines, Methedrine.
Hallucinogens LSD, Mescaline, STP, Peyote.
Cannabis derivatives Marijuana, Hashish.
Other Include tranquilizers, nonbarbiturate sedatives, glue, nutmeg, etc.

Suicidal gestures Suicidal behavior apparently without serious motivation to succeed.
Suicidal attempts Suicidal behavior apparently with serious motivation to succeed.

PERSONALITY TRAITS

This section refers to traits that are not limited to episodes of illness but are characteristic of a subject's behavior over long periods of his life. In most instances such traits will also be present during the last month. If the trait is a reason for this admission at the time of admission, in addition to being a long term problem, it should be so noted.

Rigid Uncompromising inflexibility.
Inhibited Unduly restricted in the expression of anger, disagreement or self assertion.
Histrionic Theatrical or flamboyant in the display of emotions.
Cyclothymic Alternating periods of elated mood and sadness.
Passive-aggressive Obstructing other people's goals by passive techniques, such as obstructionism, pouting, procrastination or intentional inefficiency.
Self-defeating Becoming involved in self damaging situations or doing things that result in harm to his best interests.
Dependent Difficulty coping without assistance, praise, or reassurance from others.
Aimless Tendency to have no long term goals or plans, or to keep changing them.
Hostile Overt antagonism, anger, and resentment.
Assaultive Physical acts of violence against a person.
Suspicious Mild distrust to feelings of persecution.
Domineering Attempts to exercise arbitrary or overbearing control.
Eccentric Odd or idiosyncratic behavior.
Hypersensitive (to others) Undue sensitivity to how people treat him, in that feelings are easily and often hurt, or for no good reason he feels slighted or criticized.
Tending to blame others for his difficulties when the circumstances indicate his own involvement.

Traits which may be positive or negative

Pleasure out of life Pleasure and satisfaction in activities, relationships or interests.
Involvement in voluntary leisure time activities Consider level of interest and participation. Include hobbies, or other activities not necessitated by work or social roles.
Responsible Can be depended upon to fulfill obligations necessitated by his relationship to his family, friends or associates, and to avoid actions harmful to them.
Concern for others Caring about the feelings, needs and condition of other people.
Ability to cope with stress Consider effectiveness when confronted with stressful situations, and ability to adapt to changes in life circumstances.
Judgment Ability to correctly evaluate the probable consequences of his actions.
Ambitious Desire to achieve greater status, recognition or power. Do not consider worthiness of goal.
Perseverance Persistence in attempting to achieve a goal despite obstacles. Do not consider worthiness of goal.

ARRESTS

Number Include all arrests, even if not for types noted.

PREVIOUS EPISODES

Consider all previous clearly demarcated, distinctive, and separate periods of psychopathology. The periods before and after the episode(s) need not have been free of psychopathology.

OVERALL SEVERITY OF ILLNESS

For each time period consider all evidence of psychopathology and level of impairment. Do not include prognosis.
Overtly psychotic Note if he was overtly psychotic for any length of time during the time period. The qualifying phrase "overt" is used to limit the use of the term to situations where there would be little disagreement between clinicians, e.g. the presence of marked impairment in reality testing (e.g. delusions or hallucinations), thinking, or language (e.g. incoherence).

Age when first demonstrated significant impairment because of psychopathology Give best estimate if there was no clear-cut onset of significant impairment.

Mental Status Forms

NONCOMPUTERIZED FORM

I. General Appearance. Describe the patient's dress, physical appearance, posture, gait, and facial expression.

II. Attitude During the Interview. Describe the patient's response to the interviewer.

III. Description of Thought Processes. Describe the rate of flow of thought and its continuity. Explicitly comment on looseness of associations, circumstantiality, tangentiality, perseveration, irrelevance, and incoherence. Does he block, use neologisms, exhibit echolalia, have difficulty concentrating, or have racing thoughts?

IV. Activity Level. Is the patient calm, agitated, retarded in motion, hyperactive, etc.? Note any evidence of compulsive behavior or rituals or any bizarre or idiosyncratic behavior.

V. Concept Formation. Is the patient able to abstract? (Use of proverbs may be helpful.) How much insight does he have into his own behavior?

VI. Delusions and Self-referential Thinking. Describe any delusional systems the patient may have as well as any ideas of reference (e.g., paranoid, grandiose).

VII. Phobias. Does the patient have any phobias, and if so, to what degree do they interfere in his daily functioning?

VIII. Hypochondriacal Ideation. Does the patient have any somatic complaints that do not have a basis in reality?

IX. Hallucinations and Illusions. Describe the character and content of the hallucination (e.g., visual, auditory, tactile, taste). Under what circumstances do they occur and how long do they continue?

X. Mood and Affect. Describe the patient's predominant mood (e.g., depression, elation) and affect (e.g., anger, anxiety). Is the affect inappropriate or absent? Is the patient warm or likable?

XI. Ambivalence. If remarkably present, give an illustration.

XII. Depersonalization and Derealization. Does the patient ever feel apart from himself or see himself as an actor on a stage? Does he ever feel unreal or that he does not really exist? (Has he ever done anything like cut himself to see if he does exist?)

XIII. Orientation. Does the patient know his name, the date, where he is?

XIV. Disorders of Memory. Comment on both past and present memory.

XV. General Intelligence Level. Give some rough indication of the person's intelligence. This may be facilitated by having him perform simple arithmetical problems or subtract serial sevens.

COMPUTERIZED FORM*

*Mental Status Examination Record (Form M S 9 (9/70)) Reproduced by permission of Robert L. Spitzer, M.D. and Jean Endicott, Ph.D.

Form MS9 (9/70)

MENTAL STATUS EXAMINATION RECORD (MSER)*
Read instructions on reverse side.   Page 1 of 4

Patient's last name	First name	M.I.	Facility	Ward

IDENTIFICATION

Case or consecutive number

:0: :1: :2: :3: :4: [ ] :5: :6: :7: :8: :9:
:0: :1: :2: :3: :4: [ ] :5: :6: :7: :8: :9:
:0: :1: :2: :3: :4: [ ] :5: :6: :7: :8: :9:
:0: :1: :2: :3: :4: [ ] :5: :6: :7: :8: :9:
:0: :1: :2: :3: :4: [ ] :5: :6: :7: :8: :9:
:0: :1: :2: :3: :4: [ ] :5: :6: :7: :8: :9:

Facility code

:0: :1: :2: :3: :4: [ ] :5: :6: :7: :8: :9:
:0: :1: :2: :3: :4: [ ] :5: :6: :7: :8: :9:
:0: :1: :2: :3: :4: [ ] :5: :6: :7: :8: :9:

Rater code

:0: :1: :2: :3: :4: [ ] :5: :6: :7: :8: :9:
:0: :1: :2: :3: :4: [ ] :5: :6: :7: :8: :9:
:0: :1: :2: :3: :4: [ ] :5: :6: :7: :8: :9:

Last day of week being evaluated

Jan	Feb	Mar	Apr	May	Month	Jun	Jul	Aug	Sep	Oct
1	69	70	71	72	Year	73	74	75	Nov	Dec
2	3	4	5	6		7	8	9	10	11
12	13	14	15	16	Day	17	18	19	20	21
22	23	24	25	26		27	28	29	30	31

Sex of the patient

male   female

Patient's age

:0: :1: :2: :3: :4: :5: :6: :7: :8: :9:
:0: :1: :2: :3: :4: :5: :6: :7: :8: :9:

TRANSACTION

initial evaluation   reeval-uation   partial reeval   correction   deletion

ATTITUDE TOWARD RATER

[unknown]

very positive | positive | neutral | ambivalent | negative | very negative

RELIABILITY AND COMPLETENESS OF INFORMATION

very good | good | only fair | poor | very poor

Barriers to communication or reliability were due to

refuses information	massive denial	dialect or foreign language
physical illness	preoccupation	lack of response
sensorial or cognitive disorder	conscious falsification	deafness

quality of speech

APPEARANCE

Patient looks   his age | older | younger | good looking

Apparent physical health   very good | good | only fair | poor | very poor

Physical deformity   slight | mild | mod | mark

Weight   underweight | average | overweight | gaining | losing

Height   very short | short | average | tall | very tall

Ambulation disturbance   walks with assistance | must use wheel chair | bed-ridden

Dress and grooming

	slight	mild	mod	mark
Unkempt	:2:	:3:	:4:	:5:
Inappropriate	:2:	:3:	:4:	:5:
Seductive	:2:	:3:	:4:	:5:
Neat and appropriate for occasion				

Posture		slight	mild	mod	mark
	Stooped	:2:	:3:	:4:	:5:
	Stiff	:2:	:3:	:4:	:5:
	Bizarre	:2:	:3:	:4:	:5:
Face	Impassive	:2:	:3:	:4:	:5:
	Tense	:2:	:3:	:4:	:5:
	Perplexed	:2:	:3:	:4:	:5:
	Suspicious	:2:	:3:	:4:	:5:
	Angry	:2:	:3:	:4:	:5:
	Sullen	:2:	:3:	:4:	:5:
	Bored	:2:	:3:	:4:	:5:
	Worried	:2:	:3:	:4:	:5:
	Sad	:2:	:3:	:4:	:5:
	Tearful	:2:	:3:	:4:	:5:
	Elated	:2:	:3:	:4:	:5:
	Silly	:2:	:3:	:4:	:5:
	Grimacing	:2:	:3:	:4:	:5:
	Hypervigilant	:2:	:3:	:4:	:5:

Facial expression unremarkable

Eyes		occasional	often	very often	most of time
	Avoids direct gaze				
	Stares into space				
	Glances furtively				

Set no. 0018689 [ ]   Mark last 3 digits of Set number in area below.

:0: :1: :2: :3: :4: :5: :6: :7: :8: :9:
:0: :1: :2: :3: :4: :5: :6: :7: :8: :9:
:0: :1: :2: :3: :4: :5: :6: :7: :8: :9:

*Developed by Robert L. Spitzer, M.D., and Jean Endicott, Ph.D., Biometrics Research, N.Y.S. Department of Mental Hygiene, with the assistance of the Multi-State Information System for Psychiatric Patients Project. Supported by N.Y.S. Department of Mental Hygiene, C29820 and NIMH Grants 14934 and 08534.

IBM M62389

MSER 1b

PURPOSE

The purpose of the Mental Status Examination Record (MSER) is to enable a rater to record the results of a mental status examination. Proper use of this form encourages the rater to consider all of the items on the MSER when conducting his examination. The recorded information can be used by a computer to produce a narrative description of the results of the examination. In addition, it will also be possible to use the information for the systematic evaluation of individual patients and for studies of groups of patients.

The rater may add narrative comments to the clinical record for any information for which there are no items on the form.

DATA SOURCE

The data upon which the judgments are based should be mainly from direct contact with the patient; however, other information available to the rater, such as nurses' reports or personal observation of the patient on the ward, should be used.

TIME PERIOD

The evaluation covers behavior and symptoms which occurred during the week prior to and including the day of evaluation whether the evaluation is done on admission or at a later time.

ITEMS OF INFORMATION

Some items must be marked for all patients. These items are printed in **bold type** and contain a category indicating no pathology. For example:

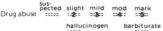

Psychomotor none slight mild mod mark
retardation

All of the remaining items are marked only when applicable for the patient being evaluated. These items should be left blank if there is no information or if there is no psychopathology. Examples are:

sus-
pected slight mild mod mark
Drug abuse

hallucinogen barbiturate

Note that a shaded line, linking a series of terms in an item requiring a scaled judgment, indicates that the rater should select no more than one term from the list.

All scaled judgments of severity should take into account how intense the behavior was as well as how much of the time it was present during the week. Thus, the ratings are a weighted average for the entire week and not necessarily the highest intensity exhibited at any one time. When making these judgments, the rater should think of the full range of the behavior that people sometimes exhibit.

NOTING JUDGMENTS

Note all judgments with a No. 2 pencil. Make a heavy dark mark between the lines of the grids. Example: ━━ To change a judgment, completely erase the incorrect mark. In filling out **IDENTIFICATION** section and **Set number**, numbers should be written in the boxes as well as noted in the grids. The numbers read from top to bottom so that the last digit is in the bottom row. If the number has fewer digits than the number of rows alloted, one or more of the top rows are left blank.

SET NUMBER

Each page of the MSER is preprinted with a seven digit Set number. The last three digits of this number are used to link the four pages together for data processing. Be sure to mark the last three digits from the Set number on all four pages.

PRINTOUT

The computer printout will contain in a narrative all of the information that the rater has noted. This will include information based on ratings of "none" as well as positive indications of psychopathology.

If a rater fails to mark an item that is supposed to be completed for all patients, the printout will note that information for this item is missing. Inconsistencies between ratings will also be indicated.

DEFINITIONS AND INSTRUCTIONS for sections and items which may be unclear.

IDENTIFICATION

Rater code Code number for person completing this form.

Last day of week being evaluated The last day of the one week being evaluated. Not necessarily the same as date the form is completed.

TRANSACTION

Initial evaluation for first time entire form used for this admission.
Reevaluation for subsequent use of entire form.
Partial reevaluation Entry of IDENTIFICATION and one or more sections of the form to indicate a change in patient's condition since the last entry. The printout will be limited to those sections.
Correction To make a correction in a previously submitted form, because of clerical or judgmental error, or new information, correct old form or completely fill out a new form. The case or consecutive number and date in the IDENTIFICATION section must be identical to the previously submitted form. The previously submitted form will be completely replaced in the file by the new form.
Deletion To delete from the file a previously submitted form, e.g. wrong case or consecutive number, wrong date, or duplicate record. Form requesting deletion must have identical case or consecutive number and date in IDENTIFICATION section as record to be deleted.

ATTITUDE TOWARD RATER

Unknown as might be the case with a mute patient.
Ambivalent At times positive, at other times, negative.
Neutral No particular emotional reaction.

RELIABILITY AND COMPLETENESS OF INFORMATION

Rater's overall judgment of accuracy and completeness of information. Example: a mute catatonic would not give information about the content of his thoughts, thereby lowering the completeness of the overall information.
Barriers to communication or reliability were due to the specific reason(s) listed.

   Quality of speech Any disturbance of speech listed later under "Quality of speech and thought" which is a barrier to communication.
   Preoccupation Exclusive focus on a topic or thought so that inadequate information is given on other topics.
   Massive denial Extensive use of the defense mechanism of denial where aspects of external reality are not acknowledged so as to avoid anxiety, as distinguished from lying which is conscious.
   Lack of response Failure to reply to questions.
   Sensorial or cognitive disorder Any disturbance listed under "Sensorium" or "Cognitive functions" which is a barrier to communication.

APPEARANCE

Apparent physical health Outward appearance of health.
Physical deformity Visibility of physical deformity causing disfigurement.
Dress and grooming Clothing, hair, makeup, jewelry, accessories.
   Unkempt Untidy or dirty.
   Inappropriate Odd or eccentric or unsuitable for the occasion.
Posture
   Stiff Holding body rigidly.
   Bizarre Odd or eccentric.
Face Facial expression. It need not be consistent with "General attitude and behavior," as with a patient who looks angry but does not act angry.
   Impassive Expressionless. When marked may be like a "zombie."
   Grimacing Distorted facial expression.
   Hypervigilant Excessive watchfulness and attentiveness, as staring closely at interviewer.
Eyes
   Glances furtively Looks about quickly and surreptitiously.

Form MS9 (9/70)
MSER

MOTOR BEHAVIOR

	none	slight	mild	mod	marked

Psychomotor retardation   none slight mild mod marked

catatonic stupor   catatonic rigidity   waxy flexibility

Psychomotor excitement   none slight mild mod marked

catatonic excitement

Tremor   slight mild mod marked

Tics

Posturing

Pacing

Fidgeting

Gait   Unsteadiness

Rigidity

Slowness

Motor abnormality possibly because of
medication   orthopedic problem   neurological disorder

GENERAL ATTITUDE AND BEHAVIOR

Positive characteristics
helpful   responsible   good sense of humor
cheerful   pleasant   likeable

Uncooperative   none slight mild mod marked

Withdrawn

Inappropriate

Impaired functioning in goal directed activities

Suspicious

Anger (overt)
sarcastic   critical   argumentative
sullen   assaultive   physically destructive
irritable   threatens violence

Provokes anger   slight mild mod marked

Suicidal behavior   none at least threats at least gesture(s) attempt(s)

Self mutilation (degree of disfiguring)   slight mild mod marked

Antisocial

Impulsive

Passive

Dependent

Domineering

Guarded

Complaining

Ritualistic

GENERAL ATTITUDE AND BEHAVIOR (continued)

	slight	mild	mod	mark

Obsequious

Despondent

Apathetic

Fearful

Dramatic

Sexually seductive

Homosexual behavior

Alcohol abuse   suspected

Drug abuse   suspected
hallucinogen   barbiturate   stimulant
narcotic   other

MOOD AND AFFECT

	none	slight	mild	mod	mark

Depression

Anxiety   with episodes of panic

Anger

Euphoria

Anhedonia

Loneliness

Quality of mood and affect   none slight mild mod mark

Flatness

Inappropriate

Lability

Diurnal mood variation   worse in morning   worse in evening

QUALITY OF SPEECH AND THOUGHT

Voice   shouts   screams
very loud   monotonous   overly dramatic
whining   very soft

Rate   very slow slow average fast very fast

Productivity   markedly reduced reduced average increased markedly increased

Incoherence   none slight mild mod mark

Irrelevance

Evasiveness

Blocking

Set no. 0018688   Mark last 3 digits of Set number in area below.

0 1 2 3 4   5 6 7 8 9
0 1 2 3 4   5 6 7 8 9
0 1 2 3 4   5 6 7 8 9

IBM M62391

MSER 2b

MOTOR BEHAVIOR
Characteristics of bodily movements that are observable.
Psychomotor retardation Generalized slowing down of physical reactions and movements.
> **Catatonic stupor** Marked decrease in reactivity to environment and reduction of spontaneous movements and activity. May appear to be unaware of nature of surroundings.
> **Catatonic rigidity** Maintaining a rigid posture against efforts to move him.
> **Waxy flexibility** Maintaining postures into which he is placed.

Psychomotor excitement Generalized overactivity.
> **Catatonic excitement** Apparently purposeless and stereotyped, excited motor activity not influenced by external stimuli.

Tics Involuntary, brief, recurrent, movements involving a relatively small segment of the body.
Posturing Voluntary assumption of an inappropriate or bizarre posture.

GENERAL ATTITUDE AND BEHAVIOR
The attitude and behavior that the patient displays in his interaction with others. This may or may not be consistent with "Content of speech and thought." For example: he may be physically assaultive but not indicate or acknowledge thoughts of doing violence to others.
Withdrawn Avoidance of contact or involvement with people.
Inappropriate Behavior that is odd, eccentric or not in keeping with the situation. Examples: exposing self, talking to self, frequent giggling.
Impaired functioning in goal directed activities Impairment in work (if work was expected) or in other goal directed activities, e.g. chores, leisure time activities, or getting dressed.
Suspicious From mild distrust to feelings of persecution. May be markedly suspicious and yet not delusional.
Anger (overt) Overall rating of overt expression of anger. Inferences of unconscious anger should not be used in making this rating.
> **Assaultive** Physical violence against a person.
> **Physically destructive** Destroys or breaks things.

Provokes anger Attitude or behavior that provokes anger in others, e.g. teases, touches others, argumentative.
Suicidal behavior As distinguished from suicidal thoughts. Include evaluation of threat to life and seriousness of intent.
Self mutilation Disfigurement resulting from deliberate damage to the body (not associated with a suicide attempt).
Antisocial Antisocial attitude or behavior, e.g. lying, encouraging breaking of rules, stealing, complacent attitude towards his own or others' antisocial behavior.
Impulsive Acts immediately without reflection.
Passive Permits himself to be acted upon without his making efforts to control the course of events.
Dependent Seeks undue assistance, praise or reassurance from others.
Domineering Examples: tries to control interview, orders others around.
Guarded Acts in a defensive or protective manner, e.g. reluctant to give information.
Ritualistic Displays compulsions or other repetitive stereotyped behavior that is not directly adaptive, e.g. hand washing rituals, endless recheckings, formalized procedures for eating or dressing.
Obsequious Servile attentiveness or marked inclination to please.
Despondent Acts discouraged, dejected, or depressed.
Apathetic Lack of feeling, interest, concern or emotion.
Dramatic Artificiality of action with exaggerated emotionalism.
Homosexual behavior Overt homosexual approaches or acts as distinguished from homosexual thoughts.
Alcohol abuse Use of alcohol during the past week which is excessive, causes physical symptoms, causes alteration in mood or behavior, or interferes with performance of expected daily routine or duties.
Drug abuse Excessive self medication; unprescribed use of drugs with effects as described above for alcohol abuse.

MOOD AND AFFECT
Emotion or feeling tone that is either observable or reported by the patient. This may or may not be consistent with the content of speech, e.g. looks sad and tearful but says he is not depressed. Inferences based on psychodynamic formulations should not be used in making these ratings, e.g. unconscious anger because the patient is overly polite.
Depression Sadness, worthlessness, failure, hopelessness, remorse, or loss.
Anxiety Apprehension, worry, nervousness, tension, fearfulness, or panic.
> **With episodes of panic** Circumscribed periods of intense anxiety.

Euphoria Exaggerated feeling of well being, not consonant with circumstances.
Anhedonia Absence of pleasure in activities that ordinarily would be pleasurable.
Flatness Generalized impoverishment of emotional reactivity, often described as "emotionally dull," or "unresponsive."
Inappropriate Affect is not appropriate for situation or is incongruous with content of speech, e.g. giggles during interview, cheerful while discussing threats to his life.
Lability Unstable emotions that shift rapidly without adequate control, e.g. sudden bursts of anger or crying.
Diurnal mood variation Consistent change in mood from morning to evening.

QUALITY OF SPEECH AND THOUGHT
Voice monotonous Lack of normal variation in pitch.
Rate Rapidity of speech and thought.
Productivity The amount of speech.
Incoherence Impairment in the form of speech which makes it difficult to understand or follow. (A bizarre delusional belief may be explained in a coherent manner.)
Irrelevance Content of remarks is not related to questions being asked or topic under discussion.
Evasiveness Deliberately avoids answering questions directly.
Blocking Sudden cessation in the train of thought or in the middle of a sentence. The patient is unable to explain the reason for the sudden stoppage.

Form MS 9 (9/70)

MSER
Page 3 of 4

QUALITY OF SPEECH AND THOUGHT (continued)

	slight	mild	mod	marked
Circumstantiality	2	3	4	5
Loosening of associations	2	3	4	5
Obscurity	2	3	4	5
Concreteness	2	3	4	5

Other

echolalia	clang associations	neologisms
flight of ideas	excessive profanity	plays on words
persever-ation	unintelligible muttering	suggestive of neurological disorder

CONTENT OF SPEECH AND THOUGHT

	unknown	none	slight	mild	mod	marked
Grandiosity	7	1	2	3	4	5
Suicidal ideation	7	1	2	3	4	5
Ideas of reference	7	1	2	3	4	5
Bizarre thoughts	7	1	2	3	4	5
Phobia(s)	7	1	2	3	4	5
Compulsion(s)	7	1	2	3	4	5
Obsession(s)	7	1	2	3	4	5

	slight	mild	mod	marked
Guilt	2	3	4	5
Alienation	2	3	4	5
Pessimism	2	3	4	5
Distrustfulness	2	3	4	5
Self pity	2	3	4	5
Inadequacy	2	3	4	5
Diminished interest	2	3	4	5
Indecisiveness	2	3	4	5
Isolation	2	3	4	5
Helplessness	2	3	4	5
Failure	2	3	4	5
Loss	2	3	4	5
Self derogatory	2	3	4	5
Resentful of others	2	3	4	5
Death	2	3	4	5
Loss of control	2	3	4	5

Harm	being harmed by others	doing harm to others
Sexual symptoms	frigidity	homosexual impulses
	potency disturbance	fears of homosexuality

Delusions	absent	unknown	suspected	likely	definite

	slight	mild	mod	marked
Persecutory delusions	2	3	4	5
Somatic delusions	2	3	4	5
Delusions of grandeur	2	3	4	5

CONTENT OF SPEECH AND THOUGHT (continued)

	slight	mild	mod	mark
Religious delusions	2	3	4	5
Delusions of guilt	2	3	4	5
Delusions of influence	2	3	4	5
Nihilistic delusions	2	3	4	5

	very little	considerable	marked
Influence of delusion on behavior			

SOMATIC FUNCTIONING AND CONCERN

	very poor	poor	normal	excessive	very excessive
Appetite					

	requires urging to eat	requires help to eat

	very easily fatigued	easily fatigued	normal	very energetic	extremely energetic
Energy level					

	sleeps excessively				feels little need for sleep
Change in sexual interest or activity	marked decrease	slight decrease	slight increase	marked increase	

Insomnia (overall severity any type)	none	slight	mild	mod	mark
	1	2	3	4	5

difficulty falling asleep	early morning awakening	awakening during night

	occa-sionally	often	very often	most of time
Incontinence				

	one	several	daily	several per day
Seizures (this week)				

	likely hysterical	likely organic
Severe sensory impairment (organic)	visual	hearing

	suspected	likely	definite
Conversion reaction			
Type	hearing loss		visual defect
paralysis	anesthesia		paresthesia
abnormal movements	pain		

Psychophysiologic reactions	none	slight	mild	mod	mark
	1	2	3	4	5
Type	upset stomach				diarrhea
consti-pation	palpitations				hyperventilation syndrome
headache	back-ache				urinary frequency
sweating	itching				

Unwarranted concern with physical health	none	slight	mild	mod	mark
	1	2	3	4	5

PERCEPTION

Hallucinations	absent	unknown	suspected	likely	definite

	slight	mild	mod	marked	un-formed	formed
Visual	2	3	4	5		
Auditory	2	3	4	5	voices	noises
Olfactory	2	3	4	5		
Gustatory	2	3	4	5		
Tactile	2	3	4	5		
Visceral	2	3	4	5		

Set no. 0018688

Mark last 3 digits of Set number in area below.

0	1	2	3	4		5	6	7	8	9
0	1	2	3	4		5	6	7	8	9
0	1	2	3	4		5	6	7	8	9

IBM M62393

MSER 3b

Circumstantiality Proceeding indirectly to goal idea with many tedious details and parenthetical and irrelevant additions.
Loosening of associations Saying things in juxtaposition which lack a logical or inherent relationship, e.g. "I'm tired. All people have eyes."
Obscurity Lack of precision and clarity.
Concreteness A tendency to deal with concepts at a sensory or partial level at the expense of considering general relationships or abstractions, e.g. literal interpretation of proverbs.
Echolalia Repetition by imitation of phrases or words said in their presence.
Clang associations Combining unrelated words or phrases because they share similar sounds, e.g. "I'm sad, mad, bad."
Neologisms Invention of new words.
Flight of ideas Abrupt and rapid changes of topic of conversation so that ideas are not completed.
Plays on words Inappropriate rhyming or punning.
Perseveration Repetition of a single response or idea in reply to various questions or repetition of words or phrases over and over in a mechanical manner.
Suggestive of neurological disorder Impairment in articulation such as those seen in various neurological disorders or expressive aphasia.

CONTENT OF SPEECH AND THOUGHT

The items in this section are descriptive of what the patient says or is thinking about. It may not be in keeping with his attitude and general behavior. For example, he may not act "dependent" yet reports feelings of "helplessness." The information may be offered spontaneously or only after questioning.

Grandiosity Inflated appraisal of his worth, contact, power or knowledge. (A patient may be markedly grandiose and yet not have delusions of grandeur.)
Suicidal ideation From occasional thoughts of killing himself, to preoccupation with method of killing himself.
Ideas of reference Detection of personal reference in seemingly insignificant remarks, objects, or events, e.g. interprets a person's sneeze as a message. (Patient may recognize absurdity of thought.)
Bizarre thoughts Content of thinking is odd, eccentric or unusual (but not necessarily delusional), e.g. preoccupation with flying saucers.
Phobia Irrational fear of a specific object or situation, e.g. fear of crowds, heights, animals; to be distinguished from free floating anxiety or fears of general conditions (getting sick, business failure).
Compulsion An insistent, repetitive, unwanted urge to perform an act which is contrary to his ordinary conscious wishes or standards, e.g. hand washing compulsion.
Obsession Persistent, unwanted thoughts which occur against his resistance, the content of which he regards as senseless, e.g. thoughts of killing child.
Alienation Feelings of estrangement, e.g. wonders who he really is, feels he is different from everybody.
Isolation Feelings of social isolation, rejection, or discomfort with people; preference for being alone.
Loss Feelings or theme of no longer having some person or object of great importance.
Self derogatory Reproaches self for things he has done or not done.
Being harmed by others Thinks of people as mistreating him, as taking advantage of him or as harming him in some way.
Frigidity Impaired pleasure from sexual intercourse.
Fears of homosexuality Fears of homosexual seduction or fears that he is a homosexual.
Potency disturbance Difficulty maintaining an erection during intercourse.
Homosexual impulses Speaks of his homosexual impulses.
Delusions Conviction in some important personal belief which is almost certainly not true.
   Persecutory delusions Examples: believes an organized conspiracy exists against him, or that he has been attacked, harassed, cheated or persecuted or that people talk about him or stare at him, when the circumstances make it almost certainly not true.
   Somatic delusions Conviction about his body that is almost certainly not true, e.g. body is rotting, someone is in his brain.

Delusions of grandeur Claims power or knowledge beyond the bounds of credibility, e.g. has special relation to God; can read people's minds.
Religious delusions A delusion involving a religious theme.
Delusions of guilt Belief that he has done something terrible or is responsible for some event or condition which is almost certainly not true, e.g. has ruined family by his bad thoughts.
Delusions of influence Claims his thoughts, mood, or actions are controlled or mysteriously influenced by other people or by strange forces.
Nihilistic delusions Believes the world is destroyed or that he or everyone is dead.
Influence of delusion on behavior The extent to which the delusional belief influences his behavior. To be left blank if patient is not delusional or if his delusion has virtually no effect on how he interacts with others or how he organizes his life.

SOMATIC FUNCTIONING AND CONCERN

Energy Level Capacity to sustain effort without fatigue. The effort may not be goal directed as with the extremely energetic manic.
Change in sexual interest or activity To be left blank if there is no change from the usual level.
Insomnia Overall rating of difficulty sleeping.
Incontinence Inability to restrain, within normal limits, the natural evacuation of the bladder or bowels.
Seizures A sudden attack of motor or sensory disturbance often involving a disturbance of consciousness.
   Likely hysterical Judged to be on a psychological basis.
   Likely organic Judged to be due to some structural or biochemical abnormality of the brain.
Severe sensory impairment (organic) Examples: blindness, deafness on a physical basis.
Conversion reaction A disturbance of the special senses or of the voluntary nervous system, often expressing emotional conflict in a symbolic manner; to be distinguished from psychophysiologic disorders which are mediated by the autonomic nervous system, from malingering which is done consciously, and from neurological lesions which cause anatomically circumscribed symptoms. Symptoms should not be listed unless they are considered conversion reactions. ("Hysterical hallucinations" should not be noted here but rather under "Perception.")
   Anesthesia Absence of sensation, generally of the skin.
   Paresthesia Perverted sense of touch, e.g. tingling, burning, tickling caused by tactile stimulus.
   Abnormal movements Examples: tremors, tics, seizures, ataxic gait.
Psychophysiologic reactions Physical symptoms usually mediated by the autonomic nervous system, and clearly caused by emotional factors. The physiological changes are those that normally accompany certain emotional states, are generally reversable and therefore do not involve permanent tissue alteration.
   Upset stomach Do not include diarrhea or constipation even if the subject refers to these symptoms as "upset stomach."
   Hyperventilation syndrome Overbreathing which may cause such symptoms as breathlessness, dizziness, paresthesias and feelings of pressure in the chest.
Unwarranted concern with physical health Concern with physical health that is apparently not warranted by actual physical condition. Include concern with one organ (e.g. cardiac neurosis) as well as with multiple organs (hypochondriasis).

PERCEPTION

Hallucinations Sensory perceptions in the absence of identifiable stimulation occurring during the waking state whether judged to be on an organic, functional, psychotic, or hysterical basis.
   Visual hallucinations
   Unformed Visual hallucinations of unformed lights, flashes, or patterns.
   Formed Visual hallucinations of people, animals, or other recognizable things.
   Auditory hallucinations Hallucinations of sounds.
   Olfactory hallucinations Hallucinations of smell.
   Gustatory hallucinations Hallucinations of taste.
   Tactile hallucinations Hallucinations of touch.
   Visceral hallucinations Hallucinations of sensations arising within the body.

Form MS 9 (9/70)

MSER   Page 4 of 4

PERCEPTION (continued)

Content of hallucinations

threatening	accusatory	flattering
benign	religious	self derogatory
grandiose	reassuring	sexual

Conviction hallucinations real knows unreal unsure convinced

Illusions slight mild mod marked

Depersonalization 2 3 4 5

Derealization 2 3 4 5

Deja vu 2 3 4 5

SENSORIUM

Orientation disturbance too disturbed to test

	unknown	none	slight	mild	mod	marked
Time						
Place						
Person (self and others)						

Memory disturbance too disturbed to test confabulation

	unknown	none	slight	mild	mod	marked
Recent						
Remote						

Clouding of consciousness 2 3 4 5

  fluctuating continuous

Dissociation

| trance | amnesia | fugue |
| hysterical attack | other | |

COGNITIVE FUNCTIONS

Attention disturbance slight mild mod marked

Distractability 2 3 4 5

Intelligence (estimate)

| unknown | superior | bright | average | borderline | retarded |

JUDGMENT

	very good	good	only fair	poor	very poor
Family relations					
Other social relations					
Employment					
Future plans	no plans (or)	very good	good	only fair	poor	very poor

POTENTIAL FOR SUICIDE OR VIOLENCE

	unsure	not sig-nificant	low	mod	high	very high
Suicide						
Physical violence						

INSIGHT AND ATTITUDE TOWARD ILLNESS

Recognition that he is ill not applicable unknown

| very good | good | only fair | little | none | says physically ill only |

INSIGHT AND ATTITUDE TOWARD ILLNESS (continued)

Motivation for working on problem not applicable unknown

| very good | good | only fair | little | none | desires refuses treatment offered |

Awareness of his contribution to difficulties not applicable unknown

| very good | good | only fair | little | none | blames circumstances others |

OVERALL SEVERITY OF ILLNESS

not ill slight mild mod marked severe among most extreme

CHANGE IN CONDITION DURING PAST WEEK

marked improv impr stable variable worse

RATER HAS WRITTEN COMMENTS ELSEWHERE

| Signature | Date |
| | |

Set no. 0018689

Mark last 3 digits of Set number in area below.

0	1	2	3	4		5	6	7	8	9
0	1	2	3	4		5	6	7	8	9
0	1	2	3	4		5	6	7	8	9

IBM M62394

MSER 4b

Content Theme of hallucinations, including interpretation patient gives to hallucinations.
Conviction that hallucinations are real The extent to which patient is convinced that hallucinations are perceptions of real external events.
Illusions The misinterpretation or alteration of a real external sensory experience to be distinguished from hallucinations, e.g. chime of clock is heard as an insulting remark; wind is heard as someone calling name.
Depersonalization Feelings of strangeness or unreality about one's own body, e.g. feels outside of body or as if part of body does not belong to him.
Derealization Feelings of strangeness or unreality about one's surroundings, e.g. everything is dreamlike.
Deja vu A subjective feeling that an experience which is occurring for the first time has been experienced before.

SENSORIUM
Orientation disturbance
Time Does not know the year, season, month, day, or time of day.
Place Does not know where he is or in what kind of place he is.
Person (self and others) Does not know who he is or misidentifies others.
Memory disturbance General disturbance in memory not limited to a discrete time period (as with hysterical amnesia).
Recent Events of the last few hours or days.
Remote Events of several years ago.
Clouding of consciousness Disturbance in perception, attention and thought with a subsequent amnesia.
Fluctuating Intermittent returning to normal consciousness.
Continuous No return to normal consciousness.
Dissociation A psychological separation or splitting off of behavior or events from consciousness.
Trance Marked unresponsiveness to the environment, usually of sudden onset, with a degree of immobility and a dazed appearance.
Amnesia A loss of memory for a circumscribed period of time on a psychological basis; to be distinguished from a generalized memory disturbance as above.
Fugue A period of amnesia with physical flight from a stressful situation with retention of habits and skills.
Hysterical attack Marked emotional display with a strong histrionic flavor and apparent loss of contact with the environment.
Other Examples: somnambulism, automatic writing, Ganser syndrome.

COGNITIVE FUNCTIONS
Attention disturbance Inability to focus on one component of a situation. Impairment may be observed by the rater or be a subjective complaint of the patient.
Distractability Attention is too easily drawn to unimportant or irrelevant stimuli.

Intelligence (estimate) Takes into account native ingenuity as well as vocabulary, academic achievements and available IQ scores. **Superior:** IQ 120+, **Bright:** 110-119, **Average:** 90-109, **Borderline:** 70-89, **Retarded:** below 70.

JUDGMENT
Ability to evaluate alternative courses of action or to draw proper conclusions from experience.
Family relations Immediate or extended family, e.g. doesn't appreciate how his behavior upsets family.
Other social relations Example: Continually feels mistreated by strangers.
Employment Example: Unrealistic job expectations.
Future plans Note either that the patient has no plans, or note the level of judgment for plans that he does have.

POTENTIAL FOR SUICIDE OR VIOLENCE
Estimate of potential for behavior in the next few days, weeks, or month.

IBM M62395

INSIGHT — ATTITUDE TOWARD ILLNESS
Use the **not applicable** category for each item if the patient is not ill now. Use the **unknown** category if patient is ill but his insight or attitude cannot be ascertained, e.g. patient is mute.
Recognition that he is ill Realization that he has emotional, mental, or psychiatric problems or symptoms.
Motivation for working on problem in some realistic manner. May involve changing his life circumstances, attitudes, or behavior. Note whether the patient desires or refuses the treatment that is being offered.
Awareness of his contribution to difficulties Use **not applicable** if the nature of the difficulty appears to be due entirely to external influences, e.g. toxic psychosis because of febrile illness. Note if patient blames circumstances and/or other people for his difficulties.

OVERALL SEVERITY OF ILLNESS during this one week
study period. Consider all of the previous items and any other evidence of psychopathology. Do not include prognosis.

CHANGE IN CONDITION
Note the most appropriate descriptive term (e.g. marked improvement) for the past week.

RATER HAS WRITTEN COMMENTS ELSEWHERE Note if
additional comments about the patient's current condition have been recorded elsewhere in the clinical record.

The Physical Examination Form

Height: Respiratory Rate:
Weight: Blood Pressure:
Temperature: Right: Left:
Pulse:

General Appearance: Describe the patient's general appearance.

Skin: Comment on skin texture and color. Is there any evidence of cyanosis, icterus, or skin eruption? Accurately describe all scars.

Lymph Nodes: Comment on the location and size of any nodes which seem abnormal.

Head and Neck: Describe the size and shape of the patient's head. Is the neck supple? Is there any evidence of thyroid enlargement? Are the carotids symmetrical? Is there a bruit over the carotids or thyroid?

Thorax and Breasts: Is the thorax symmetrical? Is there any evidence of abnormal masses or discharge from the breasts? Does the patient exhibit gynecomastia?

Heart: Comment on rate, rhythm, and quality of heart sounds and murmurs if present. Where is the apical beat? Is a thrill or gallop present?

Lungs: Describe type of breathing, flatness or dullness to percussion, and breath sounds.

Abdomen: Describe size and contour, tenderness and rigidity, and any abnormal mass or evidence of organomegaly.

Musculoskeletal: Describe posture as well as any evidence of wasting or asymmetry of the muscles. Comment on the patient's muscle strength, tone, coordination, and gait. Perform Romberg's test. Is there any sign of muscle atrophy, fibrillations, fasciculations, or involuntary movements?

Cranial Nerves: Comment on facial symmetry, deviation of the tongue, reactivity and symmetry of the pupils, evidence of nystagmus or dysconjugate eye movements, corneal reflexes, facial sensation, gag and jaw reflexes.

Sensory: Test reactions to pin prick, touch, pressure, vibration, and temperature.

Reflexes: Test the biceps, triceps, radial, abdominal, cremasteric, knee, ankle, and plantar reflexes rating as follows: 0—Absent, 1—Diminished, 2—Normal, 3—Hyperactive, 4—Hyperactive with clonus.

Pathological Reflexes Present:

Response to Physical Examination: Comment on the patient's reaction to being examined.

Summary of Positive Physical Findings:

Diagnostic Impression:

Physician's Signature:

Date:

The Discharge Summary

1. Clinician's Name:
2. Date:
3. Initials of Patient:
4. Hospital Number:
5. Birth Date:
6. Date Admitted to Unit:
7. Source of Referral:
8. Date of Discharge from Unit:
9. Discharge Diagnosis (DSM-II):
10. Demographic Data:
11. Chief Complaint:
12. History of Present Illness:
13. Personal History:
14. Mental Status Examination on Admission:
15. Course of Evaluation and/or Treatment:
    a. Summary of all contacts
    b. Medications used:
    c. Results of diagnostic tests:
    d. Changes observed in patient or situation over the course of hospitalization:
16. Formulation:
17. Disposition:
    a. Living arrangement:
    b. Therapy plan:
18. Clinician's Signature:

REFERENCES

Aarons, Z. A. (1967) Therapeutic Abortion and the Psychiatrist. *Am. J. Psychiatry*, 124:-745–754.

Aquilera, D. C., Messick, J. M., and Farrell, M. S. (1970) *Crisis Intervention: Theory and Methodology.* St. Louis, C. V. Mosby.

Bach-Y-Rita, G., Lion, J. R., Aliment, C. E., and Ervin, F. R. (1971) Episodic Dyscontrol. A Study of 130 Violent Patients. *Am. J. Psychiatry*, 127:1473–1478.

Beck, A. T. (1967) *Depression.* New York, Harper and Row.

Beck, J.C., and Worthen, K. (1972) Precipitating Stress, Crisis Theory, and Hospitalization in Schizophrenia and Depression. *Arch. Gen. Psychiatry*, 26:123–129.

Bellak, L., Small, L. (1965) *Emergency Psychotherapy and Brief Psychotherapy.* New York, Grune and Stratton.

Bergler, E. (1970) *Money and Emotional Conflicts.* New York, International Universities Press.

Bieber, I. (1965) *Homosexuality.* New York, Vintage.

Bleuler, E. (1950) *Dementia Praecox or the Group of Schizophrenias.* New York, International Universities Press.

Brill, N. Q., and Storrow, H. A. (1960) Social Class and Psychiatric Treatment. *Arch. Gen. Psychiatry*, 3:340–344.

Brown, F. (1961) Depression and Childhood Bereavement. *Journal of Mental Sciences*, 107:734–772.

Caldwell, J. M. (1967) Military Psychiatry, in *Comprehensive Textbook of Psychiatry* (A. M. Freedman, H. I. Kaplan, H. S. Kaplan, eds.). Baltimore, William and Wilkins.

Caplan, G. (1959) *Concepts of Mental Health and Consultation.* Washington, U. S. Dept. of Health, Education, and Welfare, Children's Bureau.

Caplan, G. (1960) Patterns of Mental Disorders in Children. *Psychiatry*, 23:365–374.

Caplan, G. (1961) *An Approach to Community Mental Health.* New York, Grune and Stratton.

Caplan, G. (1961) *Prevention of Mental Disorders in Children.* New York, Basic Books.

Caplan, G. (1962) *Manual for Psychiatrists Participating in the Peace Corps Program.* Washington, Medical Program Division, Peace Corps.

Caplan, G. (1964) *Principles of Preventive Psychiatry.* New York, Basic Books.

Char, W. F., and McDermott, J. F. (1972) Abortions and Acute Identity Crises in Nurses. *Am. J. Psychiatry,* 128:952–957.

Darbonne, A. (1968) Crisis: A Review of Theory, Practice, and Research. *Int. J. Psychiatry,* 6:371–379.

Dorpat, T. L., Anderson, W. F., and Ripley, H.S. (1968) The Relationship of Physical Illness to Suicide, in *Suicidal Behaviors* (H. L. P. Resnik, ed.), Little, Brown.

Durkheim, E. (1897) *Le Suicide: Étude de Sociologie* (Suicide: A Study in Sociology.) Paris, Alcan.

Erikson, E. *Childhood and Society.* (1950) New York, W.W. Norton Co.

Farberow, N. L., and Shneidman, E. S., eds. (1965), *The Cry for Help.* New York, McGraw-Hill.

Faris, R. E. L. and Dunham, H. W. (1939) *Mental Disorders in Urban Areas.* Chicago, University of Chicago Press.

Feirstein, A., Weisman, G., and Thomas, C. (1971) A Crisis Intervention model for Inpatient Hospitalization. *Current Psychiatric Therapies,* Vol. 11 (J. H. Masserman, ed.), New York, Grune and Stratton.

Fenichel, O. (1945) *The Psychoanalytic Theory of Neurosis.* New York, W.W. Norton and Co.

Freud, S. (1925) Mourning and Melancholia in *Collected Papers, IV.* London, Hogarth Press.

Friedman, I., von Mering, O., and Hinko, E. N. (1966) Intermittent Patienthood. *Arch. Gen. Psychiatry,* 14:386–392.

Gardner, E. A., Bahn, A. K., and Mack, M. (1964) Suicide and Psychiatric Care in the Ageing. *Arch. Gen. Psychiatry,* 10:547–553.

Glass, A. J. (1954) Psychotherapy in the Combat Zone. *Am J. Psychiatry,* 110:725–731.

Goffman, E. (1961) *Asylums.* New York, Anchor.

Goldstein, K. (1959) Functional Disturbances in Brain Damage in the *American Handbook of Psychiatry,* Volume I (S. Arieti, ed.), New York, Basic Books Incorporated.

Guy, W., Gross, M., Hogarty, G. E., and Dennis, H. (1969) A Controlled Evaluation of Day Hospital Effectiveness. *Arch. Gen. Psychiatry,* 20:329–338.

Halliday, J. L. (1943) Principles of Aetiology. *Brit. J. Med. Psychol.,* 19:367–380.

Harris, H. P. (1950) Postpartal Psychotic Reactions. *Medical Surgery Journal,* 103:109–112.

Hausman, A. and Rioch, D. M. (1967) Military Psychiatry. *Arch. Gen. Psychiatry,* 16:-727–739.

Hendin, H. (1967) Suicide, in *Comprehensive Textbook of Psychiatry* (A. M. Freedman, H. I. Kaplan, eds.). Baltimore, William and Wilkins.

Hiltner, S. (1972) Theological Consultants in Hospitals and Mental Health Centers. *Am. J. Psychiatry,* 128:965–969.

Hollingshead, A. B., and Redlich, F. C. (1958) *Social Class and Mental Illness.* New York, Wiley.

Hunt, R. G. (1960) Social Class and Mental Illness: Some Implications for Clinical Theory and Practice, *Am. J. Psychiatry*, 116:1065–1069.

Jacobson, G. F. (1965) Crisis Theory and Treatment Strategy. Some Sociocultural and Psychodynamic Considerations. *J. Nerv. Ment. Dis.*, 141:209–218.

Jacobson, G., Strickler, M., and Morley, E. (1968) Generic and Individual Approaches to Crisis Intervention. *A.J.P.H.*, 58:339–342.

Janis, I. L. (1958) *Psychological Stress: Psychoanalytical and Behavioral Studies of Surgical Patients.* New York, Wiley.

Kaplan, D. M., and Mason, E. A. (1960) Maternal Reactions to Premature Birth Viewed as an Acute Emotional Disorder. *Am. J. Orthopsychiatry*, 30:539–552.

Kardiner, A. (1941) *The Traumatic Neurosis of War.* Washington, National Research Council.

Klein, D. F., and Davis, J. M. (1969) *Diagnosis and Drug Treatment of Psychiatric Disorders.* Williams and Wilkin Company, Baltimore.

Leighton, A. (1959) *My Name is Legion* Vol. I. (The Stirling County Study of Psychiatric Disorder and Sociocultural Environment), New York, Basic Books.

Leighton, D. C., Harding, J. S., Macklin, D. B., Macmillan, A. M., and Leighton, A. H. (1963) *The Character of Danger*, Vol. III (The Stirling County Study of Psychiatric Disorder and Sociocultural Environment), New York, Basic Books.

Levenstein, S., Klein, D. F., and Pollack, M. (1966) Follow-up Study of Formerly Hospitalized Voluntary Psychiatric Patients: The First Two Years. *Am. J. Psychiatry*, 122:-1102–1109.

Lewis, A. J. (1953) Points of Research into the Interaction Between The Individual and Culture in *Prospects in Psychiatric Research, The Proceedings of the Oxford Conference of the Mental Research Fund* (J. M. Tanner, ed.).

Lief, H. I., Lief, V. F., Warren, C. O., and Heath, R. C. (1961) Low Dropout Rate in a Psychiatric Clinic. *Arch. Gen. Psychiatry*, 5:200–211.

Lindemann, E. (1953) The Wellesley Project for the Study of Certain Problems in Community Mental Health in *Interrelationships Between Social Environment and Psychiatric Disorders.* New York, Milbank Memorial Fund.

Lindemann, E. (1944) Symptomatology and Management of Acute Grief. *Am. J. Psychiatry*, 101:141–148.

MacMahon, B., Johnson, S., and Pugh, T. F. (1963) Relation of Suicide Rates to Social Conditions. *Public Health Rep.*, 78:285–293.

MacMahon, B., and Pugh, T. F. Suicide in the Widowed. *Am. J. Epidem.*, 81:23–31.

Mathew, H. G., Pearson, N. G., Reda, K. L. Q., Show, D. B., Steed, G. R., Thorner, M., Jones, S., Guerrier, C. J., Eraut, C. D., McHugh, P. M., Chowdhury, N. R., Jarary, M. H., and Wallace, T. J. (1971) Acute Myocardial Infarction: Home and Hospital Treatment. *British Medical Journal*, 3:334–338.

Menninger, W. C. (1948) *Psychiatry in a Troubled World.* New York, Macmillan.

Meyerowitz, S., Satlaff, A., and Romano, J. (1971) Induced Abortion for Psychiatric Indication. *Am. J. Psychiatry*, 127:1153–1160.

Parad, H. J., ed. (1965) *Crisis Intervention: Selected Readings*, New York, Family Service Association of America.

Parad, H. J., and Caplan, G. (1965) A Framework for Studying Families in Crisis in *Crisis Intervention: Selected Readings* (H. J. Parad, ed.), New York, Family Service Association of America.

Pasamanick, B., Scarpitti, F., and Dinitry, S. (1967) *Schizophrenics in the Community.* New York, Appleton-Century-Crafts.

Porter, R. A. (1966) Crisis Intervention and Social Work Models. *Community Ment. Health J.*, 2B:13–26.

Prien, R. F., Caffey, E. M., and Klett, J. (1972) Comparison of Lithium Carbonate and Chlorpromazine in the Treatment of Mania. *Arch. Gen. Psychiatry*, 26:146–153.

Rapoport, L. (1965) The State of Crisis: Some Theoretical Considerations, in *Crisis Intervention: Selected Readings* (H. J. Parad, ed.), New York, Family Service Association of America.

Rapoport, R. (1963) Normal Crisis, Family Structure, and Mental Health. *Family Process*, 2:68–80.

Reush, J. (1953) Social Factors in Therapy in *Psychiatric Treatment*, Vol. 31 (S. B. Wortis, M. Herman, and C. C. Hare, eds.), Association for Nervous and Mental Diseases, Baltimore, Williams and Wilkins.

Robins, E., and Guze, S. B. (1970) Establishment of Diagnostic Validity in Psychiatric Illness: Its Application to Schizophrenia. *Am. J. Psychiatry*, 126:983–987.

Robins, E., Guze, S. B., Woodruff, R. A., Jr., Wanokur, G., and Munoz, R. (1972) Diagnostic Criteria for Use in Psychiatric Research. *Arch. Gen. Psychiatry*, 26:57–63.

Sainsburg, P. (1955) *Suicide in London.* London, Chapman and Hall.

Shneidman, E. S., and Farberow, N. L. (1957) *Clues to Suicide.* New York, McGraw-Hill.

Simon, N., and Senturia, A. (1966) Psychiatric Sequelae of Abortion. *Arch. Gen. Psychiatry*, 15:378–389.

Simon, N., Senturia, A., and Rothman, D. (1967) Psychiatric Illness Following Therapeutic Abortion. *Am. J. Psychiatry*, 124:59–65.

Sloane, R. B. (1969) The Unwanted Pregnancy. *New Eng. J. Med.*, 280:1206–1213.

Socarides, C. W. (1968) *The Overt Homosexual.* New York, Grune and Stratton.

Spitzer, R. L., and Endicott, J. (1971) An Integrated Group of Forms for Automated Psychiatric Case Records. *Clinical General Psychiatry*, 24:540–547.

Spitzer, R. L., and Endicott, J. (1969) Diagno II: Further Developments in a Computer Program for Psychiatric Diagnosis. *Am. J. Psychiatry*, 125:12–21.

Spitzer, R.IL., and Endicott, J. (1968) Diagno: A Computer Program for Psychiatric Diagnosis Utilizing the Differential Diagnostic Procedure. *Arch. Gen. Psychiatry*, 18:-746–756.

Social Behavior and Personality Contributions of W. I. Thomas to Theory and Social Research (E. Volkart, ed.), New York, Social Science Research Council, 1951.

Srole, L. Langner, T. S., Michael, S. T., Opler, M. K., and Rennie, T. A. C. (1962) *Mental Health in the Metropolis.* McGraw-Hill Book Co., Inc., New York.

Stanton, A., and Schwartz, M. (1954) *The Mental Hospital.* New York, Basic Books.

Stevenson, I. (1959) The Psychiatric Interview, in *The American Handbook of Psychiatry*, Vol. I, (Silvano Arieti, ed.), New York, Basic Books.

Suicide Among Youth (Public Health Service Publication No. 1971). Washington, D.C., U. S. Government Printing Office, 1969.

Sullivan, H. S. (1954) *The Psychiatric Interview.* New York, Worton.

Susser, M. (1968) *Community Psychiatry, Epidemiologic and Social Theories.* New York, Random House.

Szasz, T. S. (1959) The Communication of Distress between Child and Parent. *Brit. J. Med. Psychiatry,* 32:161–170.

Thomas, C. S., and Weisman, G. K. (1970) Emergency Planning: The Practical and Theoretical Backdrop to an Emergency Treatment Unit. *Int. J. Soc. Psychiatry,* 16:-283–287.

U.S.P.H.S. (1963) Department of Health, Education, and Welfare, N.I.M.H.: Mental Health Statistics—Current Reports, Series MHB-H-7, January, 1963.

Webster's New World Dictionary of the American Language (College edition), New York, World, 1964,

Weisman, G., Feirstein, A., and Thomas, C. (1969) Three-Day Hospitalization—A Model for Intensive Intervention. *Arch. Gen. Psychiatry,* 21:620–629.

Weissman, M., Klerman, G. L., and Paykel, E. S. (1971) Clinical Evaluation of Hostility in Depression. *Am. J. Psychiatry,* 128:41–46.

Whittington, H. G. (1970) Evolution of Therapeutic Abortion as an Element of Preventive Psychiatry, *Am. J. Psychiatry,* 126:1224–1229.

Wilder, J. F., Levin, G., and Zwerling, I. (1966) A Two-Year Follow-up Evaluation of Acute Psychotic Patients Treated in a Day Hospital. *Am. J. Psychiatry,* 122:1095–1101

Wing, J. K. (1967) Institutionalism in Mental Hospitals, in *Mental Illness and Social Process* (T. Scheff, ed.), New York, Harper and Row.

Zusman, J. (1967) Some Explanations of Changing Appearance of Psychotic Patients. *Int. Psychiatry,* 3:216–237.

INDEX

Abortion(s)
detrimental effects of, 122
need for evaluation of, 122–125
Abstracting ability, 56
Acrophobia, 56
Activity level, 53
Addiction, drug. See *Drug addiction.*
Admission(s), 14, 33–39
family interview at, 35
gathering information at, 35–37
of adolescent, 37
of attempted suicide patient, 34
of foreign patient, 34
of patient under 18 years, 34
of patient with children, 34
of patient with medical problem, 34
of psychotic, 34
of referred patient, 33
special considerations concerning, 34–35
Adolescent(s)
admission of, 37
discharge of, 38
in crisis, 120–122
living with relatives, 82
psychiatric problems of, 43
school counselors for, 82
sexual practices of, 45
social workers and, 82
Adolescent treatment program, 82
Affect
described in case history, 54
flat, 55, 57
inappropriate, 58

Affect *(continued)*
lability of, 58
Age, suicide and, 63
Agencies
outside, training programs in, 28
visited by crisis unit staff, 27
Agoraphobia, 56
Alcohol, patient use of, described in case history, 46
Alcoholic(s)
discharge of, 38
selection for crisis unit, 102
Alcoholics Anonymous, 81, 101, 103
Alcoholism
assaultive behavior and, 65
barbiturate addiction with, 101
chlordiazepoxide in, 70, 101
depression with, 103
detoxification in, 102–103
Diazepam in, 70
domestic crisis and, 105
group psychotherapy in, 80
medical complications in, 102
suicide and, 62, 64
thiamine in, 101
Ambivalence, 55, 57
Amitriptyline, 69
Amnesia, 141
Anger, displaced, 65
Anhedonia, 57
Antidepressant(s), 69–70
for geriatric patient, 128, 129
tricyclic, 68, 69–70
Antiparkinson drugs, 71

Anxiety
general appearance and, 53
in staff members, 125
phenothiazines in, 69
toleration of, by mental health
professional, 19
Apathy, 57
Appearance, general, anxiety and, 53
Assaultive behavior, 65
Association(s)
clang, 57
loose, 58
Asthma, group psychotherapy in, 80

Barbiturates, 71
addiction to, 100–102
Behavior
assaultive, 65
of mental health professional, 20
patterns of, in crisis, 4
Blocking, 57
Brain syndrome, organic, 54, 140
Butyrophenones, 68

Case history
academic development described in,
48
affect described in, 54
alcohol use given in, 46
ambivalence described in, 55
birth and early childhood described
in, 47
chief complaint described in, 44
comprehensive, 43
computerized, 43
concept formation recorded in, 56
delusions described in, 55
description of patient in, 44
drug use described in, 46, 51
family history in, 47–48, 50
financial resources described in, 45
hallucinations described in, 55
history of present illness in, 44
hypochondria described in, 56
intelligence described in, 54
interpersonal relationships described
in, 48–49
legal history in, 51
living arrangements described in, 50
medical history in, 51
military history in, 51

Case history (continued)
mood described in, 54
occupational, 49–50
of adolescent in crisis, 120–122
of alcohol detoxification, 102–103
of barbiturate addiction, 101–102
of character disorder, 135–137
of crisis therapy, 117–119
of domestic crisis, 104–106
of drug psychotic patient, 97–99
of encephalitis, 140
of evaluation for abortion, 123–125
of geriatric patient, 127–129
of grief reaction, 114–115
of homicidal patient, 107–108, 112–
113
of involutional psychosis, 95–97
of legal referral, 112–113
of manic patient, 89–91
of melodrama, 110–111
of organic brain syndrome, 140
of patient unresponsive to treatment,
140
of postpartum psychosis, 125–127
of resource-devouring patient, 132–
133
of resourceless patient, 130–131
of schizophrenic(s), 92–95, 112–113
of sociopathic patient, 133–135
of suicidal patient, 108–109
of transient situational crisis, 116
personal, 46
phobias described in, 56
psychiatric, 40, 46
psychosexual development described
in, 49
psychosocial, 40–59
functions of, 41
religious development described in,
49
sexual practices described in, 45
sleep patterns described in, 45
Character disorder, 135–137
Child-rearing, group psychotherapy in,
80
Chlordiazepoxide, 70, 101, 103
Chlorpromazine, 68, 69
Clorprothixene, 69
Church groups, referral to, 83
Circumstantiality, 57
Clang associations, 57
Claustrophobia, 56
Clergy

Clergy *(continued)*
   as consultants, 28
   on crisis team, 18, 28
   referral to, 83
Clinic(s), referral to, 83, 84
Clinicians, referring, 24, 25
Communes, referral to, 84
Community
   crisis unit relationship with, 21,
     27–29
   crisis unit staff from, 18, 27
Community agencies, referral to, 85
Compulsion(s), 57
Concept formation, 56
Concreteness, 57
Condensation, 57
Consultants, clergy as, 28
Convalescent homes, referral to, 84
Crash-pad treatment centers, 82
Crisis
   adaptive resolution of, 5
   adolescent in, 120–122
   behavior patterns in, 4
   chronic, 130–137
   definition of, 6, 22
   domestic, 104–106
   due to emotional stress, 5
   evaluation of, 37
   external stress, 114–119
   intrapsychic changes in, 5, 23
   life cycle, 120–129
   mastery of, in coping with future
     crises, 5
   therapy, 117–119
   transient situational, 116–117
   with potential for violence, 104–113
Crisis intervention
   development of technique, 3
   examples of, 87–142
   family in, 6
   generic approach to, 4
   goals in, 17
   history of, 3–9
   in combat areas, 4
   process of, 31–86
   psychosocial supports in, 6
Crisis intervention unit, 10–14
   admission to. See *Admission(s).*
   clinicians on, supervision of, 11
   community relations of, 27–29
   day's activities of, 13
   design of, 13
   director of, 10–12

Crisis *(continued)*
   duration of stay on, 73–76
   esprit de corps of, 12
   evening staff duties on, 14
   head nurse of, 12–14
   meetings of, referring clinicians at-
     tending, 28
   outpatient program of, 78, 81
   patient arrival on, 35
   patient population in, 43
   referrals made from, 81–86
   referring clinician and, 25
   relationship with community, 27–29
   selection of alcoholic patients, 102
   staff members of, anxiety in, 125
     teaching of community groups by,
      28
     visits to other hospitals, 28
     visits to outside agencies, 27
   staffing of, 27
   time schedule of, 12
   visiting hours to, 14
Crisis team, 15–21
   clergy on, 18
   community workers on, 18
   daily schedule of, 15
   goals of, 17
   group decision in, 17
   group leader of, 15
   in outpatient therapy, 74
   interchangeability of roles in, 16
   nurses on, 17
   psychiatric aides on, 18
   psychiatrist on, 18
   students on, 18
   task responsibilities of, 17
     during hospitalization, 74–76

Daytop, referral to, 81
Deculturation, 6
Dé jà vu, 57
Delusion(s), 55, 57
Depersonalization, 57
Depression
   activity level in, 53
   antidepressants in, 68, 69–70
   due to medical illness, 138
   in alcoholism, 103
   in character disorder, 135
   in geriatric patient, 127
   in grief reaction, 115
   in sociopathic patient, 133

Depression *(continued)*
  in resource-devouring patient, 132
  psychotherapy in, 70
  psychotropic agents in, 67, 69
  suicide and, 61, 64, 108, 109
Derealization, 57
Detoxification, 75, 100–103
Diagnostic problems, 138–142
Diazepam, 70
Discharge, 37–39
Discharge summaries, 86, 172
Disorientation, 53, 54
Displaced anger, 65
Domestic crisis, 104–106
Drug(s)
  history of use, in case history, 46, 51
  withdrawal from, 100–102
Drug addiction
  group psychotherapy in, 80
  suicide and, 62
Drug programs, 81
Drug psychosis, 97–99

Echolalia, 57
Echopraxia, 57
Elavil, 69
Elderly, lack of psychiatry for, 6
Emotion(s)
  crisis due to, 5
  of mental health professional, 20
Employment, for patient, 76
Encephalitis, 140
Ethnic organizations, referral to, 85
Euphoria, 57

Family
  in administering psychotropic drugs,
    68
  in crisis intervention, 6
  interview of, at admission of patient,
    35
  involvement in discharge planning,
    37–39
Family agencies, referral to, 84
Family history
  at admission, 36
  in case history, 47–48, 50
  of suicide, 64
Family physician, referral to, 83
Family system, readjustment of, 76
Family therapy, 76, 80

Finances, attitude toward, 45
Financial resources, given in case his-
    tory, 45
Flat affect, 55, 57
Flight of ideas, 58
Fluphenazine, 42, 68, 71

Gay Liberation, referral to, 85
Geriatric patient, 127–129
Grief reaction, 114–115
Group(s)
  church, referral to, 83
  support, 80

Haldol. See *Haloperidol.*
Halfway houses, referral to, 84
Hallucination(s), 55, 56, 58
Haloperidol, 69
  antiparkinson drugs with, 71
  in mania, 71, 90, 91
Hashish smoking, 97
History
  case. See *Case history.*
  medical, 58
  patient, from outside therapist, 38
  surgical, 58
Homicidal ideation
  obsessive, 66
  reduction of, 75
Homicidal patient, 106–108
  case history of, 107–108, 112–113
  hospitalization for, 66
Homicide
  evaluation of potential for, 60–66
  patient thoughts of, in case history, 46
Homosexuality, 62
Hospital(s)
  general, referral to, 84
  psychiatric, inpatient treatment at,
    83
  visits by staff members to, 28
Hospitalization
  duration of, for psychotic, 75
  episodic, 76
  long-term, detrimental effects of, 6
    reduction of, 61
  of homicidal patient, 66
  of suicidal patient, 66
  tasks of crisis unit during, 74–76
Hunger strike, 116
Hydrophobia, 56

Hypochondria
 psychophysiologic disorders versus, 57
 recorded in case history, 56
 somatic delusions versus, 57
 suicide and, 64
Hypomania
 lithium carbonate in, 71
 phenothiazines in, 69
Hysterical neurosis, 141–142
 group psychotherapy in, 80

Idea(s)
 flight of, 58
 of reference, 55
Illusion(s), 58
Imipramine, 69
Inappropriate affect, 58
Incapacitation, resolution of, 75
Insomnia
 in transient situational crisis, 116
 suicide and, 61
Institutionalism, 6
Intelligence, recorded in case history, 54
Interpersonal relationships, recorded in case history, 48–49
Involutional psychosis, 95–97

Legal history, in case history, 51
Legal organizations, referral to, 85
Lability of affect, 58
Librium, 70, 101, 103
Life cycle crisis, 120–129
Lithium therapy, 42, 71
 in manic-depression, 68, 89, 91
 indications for, 41
Loose associations, 58

Manic patient, 89–91
 activity level in, 53
 case history of, 89–91
 haloperidol for, 71, 90, 91
 lithium carbonate for, 71, 89, 91
 phenothiazines for, 69, 71
 psychotropic agents for, 67
Manic-depressive illness, lithium carbonate in, 68, 71
Marital dysharmony, 80
Marital status, suicide and, 61

Medical history
 in case history, 51
 of presenting patient, 58
Medical illness, neurosis due to, 138–139
Medication, patient acceptance of, 75
Medication groups, 80
Mellaril, 68, 69
Melodrama, 110–111
Memory disturbance, 54
Mental health centers, referral to, 82
Mental health professional, 19–21
Mental status examination, 52–58
 by nonmedical psychiatric professional, 52
 forms for, 158–169
  computerized, 161–169
  noncomputerized, 158–159
 glossary of terms used in, 57–58
 memory disturbance of patient in, 54
 patient activity level in, 53
 patient appearance in, 53
 patient disorientation in, 53
Methadone, 71
Military history, in case history, 51
Monoamine oxidase inhibitors, 70
Mood, described in case history, 54

Nardil, 70
Navane, 69
Neurosis
 due to medical illness, 138–139
 hysterical, 141–142
Nonpsychiatric clinics, referral to, 83
Nurse(s)
 head, 12–14
 task responsibilities of, 17
Nursing homes, referral to, 84

Obesity, 80
Obsession, 58
Occupation, recorded in case history, 49–50
Organic brain syndrome, 54, 140
Outpatient treatment
 by crisis unit, 74, 78, 81
 private, 81

Parnate, 70
Patient, 22–26

Patient *(continued)*
  academic development of, 48
  acceptance of medication by, 75
  acceptance of realities by, 75
  acceptance of structure by, 75
  activity level of, 53
  admission to crisis unit. See *Admission(s)*.
  affect of, 54
  ambivalence of, 55
  appearance of, 53
  arrival of, on crisis unit, 35
  attempted suicide by, 34
  attitude toward finances, 45
  case history of, 36. See also *Case history*.
  chief complaint of, 44
  concept formation by, 56
  decisions of, communication of, 74
  delusions of, 55
  description of, 44
  detoxification of, 75, 100–103
  disorientation of, 53
  disposition of, 77–86
    errors in clinical judgment on, 77
  drug use by, 51
  early childhood of, 47
  episodic hospitalization of, 76
  evaluation of, 74, 78
  family history of, 47–48, 50
  finding employment for, 76
  foreign, 34
  geriatric, 127–129
  hallucinations of, 55
  hypochondriacal, 56
  incapacitation resolved in, 75
  information about, from outside therapist, 38
  intelligence of, 54
  interpersonal relationships of, 48–49
  introduction of therapist to, 29
  lack of response to treatment, 139, 140
  legal history of, 51
  living arrangements of, 50
  manic. See *Manic patient*.
  medical evaluation of, 58–59
  medical history of, 58
  memory disturbance in, 54
  mental status examination of. See *Mental status examination*.
  mood of, 54

Patient *(continued)*
  military history of, 51
  observation of, to obtain information, 36
  occupational history of, 49–50
  phobia in, 56
  poor communication by, 41
  problems of, clarification of, 74
  psychiatric history of, 51
  psychosexual development of, 49
  psychotically disturbed. See *Psychotic patient*.
  records on, 39
  referral of, 33. See also *Referral*.
  religious development of, 49
  resource-devouring, 131–133
  resourceless, 130–131
  selection for psychotherapy, 79–81
  senile, referral to nursing and convalescent homes, 84
  sexual development of, 49
  social supports for, 41
  sociopathic, 133–135
  sources of information about, 38
  sources of referral of, 24–25
  subculture of, economic structure of, 45
  suicidal. See also *Suicide*.
    discharge of, family involvement in, 38
    episodic treatment of, 61
  suicidal thought of, questioning about, 52
  surgical history of, 58
  types of, 23
  under 18 years, admission of, 34
  with children, admission of, 34
  with medical problem, admission of, 34
Patient population, in crisis unit, 43
Perphenazine, 68
Perseveration, 58
Phenelzine, 70
Phenothiazine(s), 68–69. See also specific drug; for example, *Chlorpromazine*.
  antiparkinson drugs with, 71
  for homicidal patient, 108
  in drug psychosis, 98
  in involutional psychosis, 96
  in mania, 71
  in postpartum psychosis, 126
  in schizophrenia, 68, 92–95, 108

Phenothiazine(s) *(continued)*
  side effects of, 69, 71
Phobia(s)
  definition of, 56, 58
  group psychotherapy in, 80
  recorded in case history, 56
  types of, 56
Physical examination form, 170–171
Physical illness, suicide and, 61
Physician
  family, referral to, 83
  nonpsychiatric, referral to, 83
Postpartum psychosis, 125–127
Prolixin, 42, 68, 71
Psychiatric aides, 18
Psychiatric history, in case history, 51
Psychiatrist, 17, 18
Psychiatry, lack of, in low economic
    classes and elderly, 6
Psychomotor retardation, 58
Psychophysiologic disorders, 57
Psychosis. See also specific psychosis;
    for example, *Drug psychosis.*
  involutional, 95–97
  postpartum, 125–127
  restful sleep in, 68
Psychosocial history forms, 145–157
  computerized, 149–157
  noncomputerized, 145–148
Psychosocial supports, 6
Psychosomatic illnesses, 69
Psychotic patient, 89–99
  admission of, 34
  discharge of, 37, 38
  duration of hospitalization in, 75
Psychotherapy
  brief, 79
  emergency versus longer techniques,
    7
  forms of, 79
  group, 79–80
  in depression, 70
  innovative approaches to, 9
  long-term, 79
  selecting patients for, 79–81
Psychotropic agents, 67–72. See also
    specific agent; for example,
    Chlorpromazine.
  continued administration of, 68
  in depression, 67
  in mania, 67
  in schizophrenia, 67, 68

Race, suicide and, 64
Referral
  back to therapy, 85
  by clinicians, 25–26
  combined, 85
  evaluation, by nonpsychiatrists, 29
  information obtained at admission,
    33
  lack of, 85
  legal, 112–113
  sources of, 24–25
  to Alcoholics Anonymous, 81
  to clergy and church groups, 83
  to commune, 84
  to community agencies, 85
  to convalescent home, 84
  to ethnic organizations, 85
  to family agencies, 84
  to family physician, 83
  to general hospital, 84
  to halfway house, 84
  to medical inpatient facilities, 84
  to nonpsychiatric physicians or clin-
    ics, 83
  to nursing home, 84
  to outpatient follow-up, 81
  to private psychiatric hospital, 83
  to private therapist, 81
  to public psychiatric hospital, 83
  to relatives, 82
  to school clinics, 84
  to school counselors, 82
  to social workers, 82
  to work clinics, 84
Referring clinicians, at unit meetings,
    28
Rehabilitation groups, 80
Relatives, referral to, 82
Religion, suicide and, 64
Religious development, given in case
    history, 49
Retardation, psychomotor, 58

Schizophrenia
  acute, 91–93
  chronic, 93–95
    case history of, 94–95, 112–113
  classification of, 42
  home treatment of, 9
  phenothiazines in, 69, 92–95, 108
  psychotropic agents in, 67, 68

Schizophrenia *(continued)*
  suicide and, 60, 62
Schizophrenic patient, acceptance of
    structure by, 75
School clinics, referral to, 84
School counselors, 82
Senile patients, 84
Sex, suicide and, 62
Sexual development, 49
Sexual practices, 45
Sleep
  for psychotic, 68
  patterns of, 45
Social integration, 61
Social workers, 82
Socioeconomic classes, low, lack of psy-
    chiatry for, 6
Sociopathic patient, 133–135
Speech, tangential, 58
Stelazine, 68, 71
Stress
  emotional, 5
  external, 114–119
Students, on crisis team, 18
Stupor, catatonic, 57
Suicidal ideation
  in resource-devouring patient, 132
  reduction of, 75
  tricyclic antidepressants in, 70
Suicidal patient, 108–109
  acceptance of realities by, 75
  family support for, 65
  episodic treatment of, 61
Suicide
  age factors in, 63
  alcoholism and, 62, 64
  attempted, 34
  death of intimate and, 64
  depression and, 61, 64, 108, 109
  evaluation of potential for, 60–66
  family history of, 64
  homosexuality and, 62
  hypochondria and, 64
  insomnia and, 61
  lethality of attempts at, 63
  living arrangements and, 63
  marital status and, 61
  patient thoughts of, 46, 52
  physical illness and, 61

  previous attempts at, 63
  racial factors in, 64
  religious factors in, 64
  schizophrenia and, 60, 62
  sex factors in, 62
  social integration and, 61
  tendency toward, hospitalization in,
    66
Support groups, 80
Surgical history, 58
Synanon, referral to, 81

Tangential speech, 58
Taractan, 69
Thanatophobia, 56
Therapists, introduction to patient, 29
Therapy effectiveness, evaluation of, 42
Thiamine, 101
Thioridazine, 68
Thiothixene, 69
Thorazine, 68, 69
Tofranil, 69
Tranquilizer(s), phenothiazine. See
    Phenothiazine(s).
Tranylcypromine, 70
Treatment, episodic, 39
Trifluoperazine, 68, 71
Trilafon, 68

Valium, 70
Verbigeration, 58
Violence, crisis with potential for, 104–
    113
Visiting hours, 14

Wartime, crisis intervention in, 4
Welfare department, referral to, 85
Welfare Moms
  case history related to, 121
  referral to, 85
Wechsler Adult Intelligence Scale, 54
Withdrawal syndrome, with barbitu-
    rates, 100
Women's Liberation, referral to, 85
Work clinics, referral to, 84